SANDBAG HYPERTROPHY

THE COMPLETE SANDBAG TRAINING MANUAL

CODY JANKO

STREAMLINE
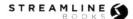
BOOKS

Sandbag Hypertrophy

The Complete Sandbag Training Manual

Published by Streamline Books

Kansas City, MO

www.streamlinebookspublishing.com

Book Cover Design by Abigael Elliott

ISBN:

979-8-89165-173-9 *Paperback*

979-8-89165-174-6 *E-book*

To Desiree for your unending love and support.

To Clover and Cash for always greeting me at the door.

To my parents for raising me to be kind.

CONTENTS

AUTHOR'S NOTE

This is a book about lifting heavy sandbags.

It's also a book about calisthenics circuits.

Mainly though it's a guide on using sandbags to make yourself big and strong.

That's what they do.

That's what they did for me.

For me, they are the axis on which everything shifted,

The turning point in my training.

Now there is only before sandbags, and after sandbags.

Before sandbags I tried just about everything there is to improve myself.

From heavy barbell deadlifts to thousand-rep bodyweight marathon sessions,

I've been working at this for a while.

Along the way I came to understand the simple truth about exercise:

Everything works.

When approached with intensity, with real honest effort, any training method will cause change.

As the author of a book on heavy sandbag training, this may seem like a strange thing for me to say.

Shouldn't I spend the next three hundred words doing my best to convince you sandbags are the ultimate training tool?

Wouldn't it be in my best interest to tell you everything that's wrong with everything that isn't a heavy sandbag?

Probably.

And I suppose I will.

But first, let me do the opposite.

As much as I'd like you to read this book, I won't intentionally mislead you.

As exciting as it may be, as much as I enjoy the motivation that comes with these kinds of stories, I can't in good conscience tell you sandbags are completely responsible for every bit of progress I've made.

It simply wouldn't be true.

Sandbags have changed me in every way shape and form, that much is certain, but I spent nearly a decade dedicated to traditional gym training (barbells, calisthenics, cables, etc.) before I ever touched a sandbag.

The basic stuff took me from a small 5 ft 8, 115 lb distance runner to someone instantly recognizable as a lifter. I added my first 30 lbs of muscle training in the traditional way, and I'll never know how things would have turned out had I worked with sandbags from the start.

What I can say is, the time I've spent lifting heavy sandbags has been the most productive of my life. They've added nearly as much muscle to my frame in nearly half the time.

There's a type of cohesiveness I have now that wasn't there before, as if every muscle looks exactly the way it's supposed to.

Like this is the shape a strong body is meant to have.

The shape taken by strong men of the past who relied on strength for survival.

Sandbags have also given me what can only be described as 'farmer strength'.

It's a type of widespread general toughness,

The strength to succeed under any circumstance,

Strength in its most fundamental shape.

Everything works, but there's nothing quite like a heavy sandbag.

For those of you out there who want more from your training, those of you ready to take the next step and discover the true power of heavy sandbag lifting, I think you'll find this book useful.

In the following chapters, you'll learn everything there is to know about lifting sandbags, down to the smallest detail.

This is a complete sandbag guide, a set of instructions you can use to transform yourself.

So if you're ready to get strong like a strongman, powerful like an Olympic weightlifter, yoked like a wrestler, tough like a rugby full-back, fit like a trail runner, and functional like a residential mover, you're in the right place.

Good luck.

-Cody

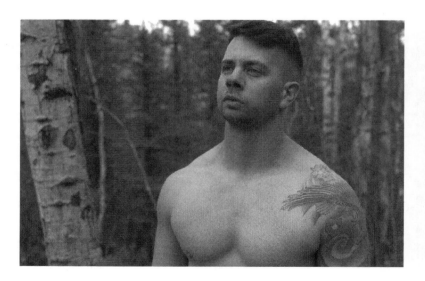

STRENGTH

What is true strength?

For some, the word 'strength' brings to mind images of giants straining to deadlift a barbell, or bodybuilders pushing beyond failure to bench just one more rep.

Others imagine strength in the shape of a one-arm pull-up, a handstand, or a planche.

I think of a day 15 years ago, the day I witnessed a feat of strength so incredible it seems taken straight from myth.

It was a Saturday in May...

A family friend was moving from one apartment to the next, and a few of us went to help carry boxes and furniture. The early 20th-century building was run down, and the elevator was out of order. Our only option was the stairwell, four flights down to the moving truck.

Many hours after arriving, countless trips up and down those stairs behind us, all that remained in the apartment was an old grand piano. At the time I think most of us just assumed the piano would stay behind. What else was there to do, it's not like someone could actually lift the thing.

Of course, the piano did need to go, just like everything else.

Among those of us helping with the move was an uncle of mine who had worked off and on as a residential mover for many years. Prior experience in mind, and because the rest of us were still young guys built more for cross-country running than for moving heavy things, it fell on him to decide what should be done with the giant instrument.

After a quick inspection, he seemed to come to a decision.

He made his way outside to his truck, returning a few minutes later with a pile of moving blankets, and what looked to be a collection of thick tow straps. A few minutes after that the piano was broken down and wrapped completely in the blankets, with the tow straps woven tightly around the outside, securing everything in place.

After double, and triple checking the straps, making certain they wouldn't come undone, he did it.

Without a moment's hesitation he flipped the piano onto one side like you would a large tire, and using the straps for support, picked it up.

He actually LIFTED the thing, making it seem no heavier than the hundred small boxes we'd moved that day.

Once the piano was off the ground, he leveraged it against his body and started down the stairs. Moving with deliberate certainty, like the slow and powerful shifting of a tectonic plate backed by a power strong enough to shape mountains he made his way down all four flights of stairs in one continuous go.

And that was that.

No moment of triumph or celebration at the end, just a smile and a wave as he hopped in his truck and left.

At the time I didn't know something like that was even possible.

"Where do you begin to lift a piano of that size?"

"How could you possibly move it from one side of a room to the other, let alone down all those stairs?"

Even after all these years the physical strength required to carry that piano far outclasses any gym lift I can think of, and the willpower to keep going after that first flight of stairs, it's completely beyond what most consider mental toughness. To my uncle, it was just another day as a residential mover, but to me it was legendary.

Since that day 15 years ago, I've come to realize I'm a bodybuilder at heart. I want to become strong, but no matter what I do, muscle will always be a priority. Strength at the expense of looking strong will never be enough. Once I accepted that basic truth, the way forward became clear, I needed to find the answer to a question.

"What can I do to make myself piano-moving strong like a residential mover, while at the same time getting big like a bodybuilder?"

It took a while, but I believe I've found that answer.

The way forward lies with a heavy sandbag and a calisthenics circuit.

SANDBAGS & CALISTHENICS

A heavy sandbag is brutal in its simplicity and makes all other forms of heavy lifting feel easy by comparison. The strength to lift a sandbag is the strength to lift anything.

A barbell.

A grand piano.

An opponent.

The sandbag gives you mastery over all of these things and more. It's a return to strength in its purest form, the modern-day equivalent to ancient man lifting stones.

Heavy sandbag lifting also gets you yoked.

Like an ox full of the power to overcome any obstacle, the sandbag gives you a body that looks STRONG. There's no other way to say it.

A thick neck.

Massive traps.

A back dense enough to make even the most seasoned body-builder envious.

Arms that speak of strength in the natural world.

A core that's so stable and defined you'll look lean and shredded even when you aren't.

Glutes and hamstrings like a power athlete.

With heavy sandbag lifting you earn the intimidating shape of one who is truly strong.

Calisthenics circuits fill in the rest, adding even more muscle to your frame and building elite strength of mind while granting you endurance on par with any athlete. A true calisthenics circuit will teach you what it means to push beyond what you thought was possible. With time, you'll reach a place few ever get to.

Together, heavy sandbag lifting and calisthenics circuits give you everything you could hope for in a training program, here's how to do it.

PROGRAMMING

With this book, you'll gain a solid understanding of how a sandbag and calisthenics training routine is set up. In addition to multiple complete training programs you can follow, at the end of each chapter will be a section on programming, detailing everything on where to place an exercise and why it goes there. This way if you decide to create your own routine, you'll know exactly where to start.

When setting up a sandbag training day, it will help to think of it as being made up of two distinct parts: power, and strength. All sandbag exercises require both, but thinking this way will improve the productivity of your workouts a great deal. Part one of the workout will be focused on both technical, and power-based movements, part two will be focused on pure strength-based movements.

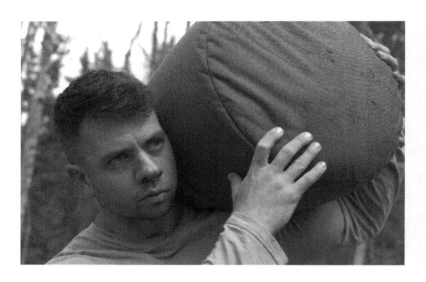

1

THE LIFT FROM THE GROUND

BEFORE YOU CAN DO anything with a sandbag you first need to get it off the ground. It's easy to rush past this part without much thought as it's less exciting than some other things, but this is a mistake. In addition to offering many unique benefits of its own, the basic lift from the ground lays the foundation for everything to come.

For most, this part of lifting a sandbag will start out as a strong point in the chain. There's not much technique involved, and raw strength is usually enough. Once you become more skilled in other areas though, it's easy to fall behind. You may, for example, shoulder heavier sandbags by improving your technique with the movement, but if you want to lift heavy things from the ground there's no getting around it, you must become stronger.

When lifting a sandbag from the ground there are three different starting positions you can use: vertical, horizontal, and standing upright. Each starting position comes with its own unique set of challenges, and you may find one suits your particular build better than the others, but they're all viable long term.

VERTICAL LIFT FROM THE GROUND

Lifting a sandbag from a vertical position on the ground is often the easiest method for beginners. With this style, your hands stay relatively close together, which allows you to maintain a more upright torso angle. This puts you at a leverage advantage and may feel more natural for some lifters.

The most difficult part of using this lifting technique is balance. To keep hold of the sandbag you must grab it directly at its center or it will fall from your hands.

The technique also comes with one major problem: heavier sandbags are usually longer, and a longer sandbag is more likely to run into your body as you try to lift it. This means that as you become stronger, the exercise becomes more difficult. Even so, the vertical lift from the ground is a great place to get started lifting sandbags.

VERTICAL LIFT FROM THE GROUND: HOW TO

To perform the vertical lift from the ground, stand directly over top of a sandbag and wedge your hands underneath each side. Take a deep breath and brace, and lift by driving your feet into the ground and extending your hips while keeping your chest held high. The sandbag should end in a vertical, standing position on your lap.

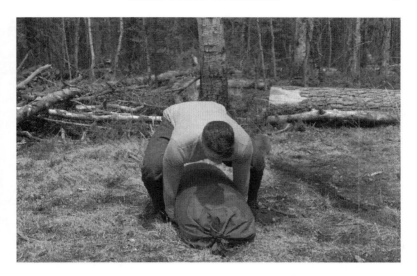

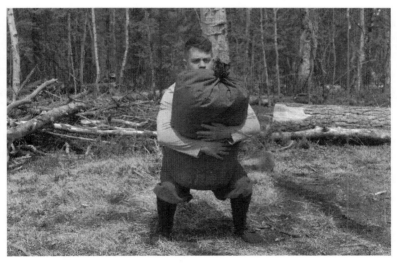

HORIZONTAL LIFT FROM THE GROUND

Lifting a sandbag from a horizontal position on the ground is the most widely used technique. It's a very intuitive approach, and is often the natural choice for anyone already familiar with barbell strength training, as the exercise more closely resembles a deadlift than the other two lifting styles.

Many elite athletes use the horizontal lift as their primary sandbag lifting technique. It has the potential to make you very strong, and should have a place in any sandbag training routine, but it's not perfect. For some lifters the exercise may eventually act as a roadblock, stalling progress in other areas. Similar to the vertical lifting technique, the difficulty of the exercise is determined by the shape of the sandbag.

We can compare this to the barbell deadlift. When lifting a barbell you'll always be stronger using a standard, shoulder-width grip than you are when using a wide, snatch grip. The snatch grip forces you to bend over further, and amplifies the difficulty. The same thing happens with sandbags. A longer sandbag means a wider grip, which means more strength is required.

HORIZONTAL LIFT FROM THE GROUND: HOW TO

To perform the horizontal lift from the ground, stand directly over top of a sandbag and wedge your hands underneath both ends, palms facing inwards towards each other, arms in a neutral position. Take a deep breath and brace, and lift the sandbag by pushing the ground away with your feet, driving your chest up, and extending your hips. The lift should end with the sandbag resting horizontally on your lap.

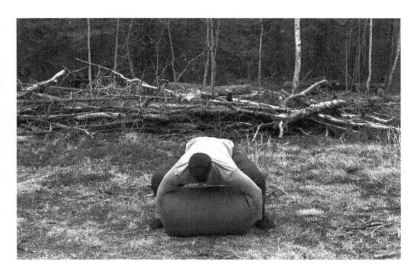

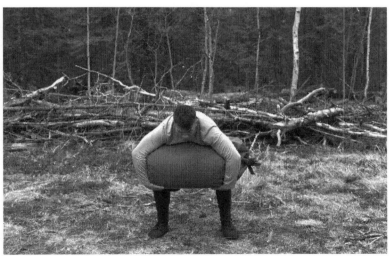

STANDING UPRIGHT LIFT FROM THE GROUND

The final way to lift a sandbag is from an upright standing position. This method takes more skill to master and doesn't work very well with smaller sandbags, but once you start lifting heavier weights it can feel almost like a cheat code.

The problem with the vertical, and horizontal lifting techniques is difficulty scaling. With those lifting styles, a longer sandbag is more difficult to lift. The lift from an upright standing position works in the opposite way. A longer sandbag stands taller, which lowers the difficulty. This makes the upright lifting technique the preferred method for many advanced lifters.

STANDING UPRIGHT LIFT FROM THE GROUND: HOW TO

The lift from an upright standing position has two distinct variations:

Variation 1: Wrap your arms around the sandbag with a bear hug grip, somewhere around three quarters of the way up. Take a deep breath and brace, and squeeze the sandbag as hard as you can, hugging it to your chest. Lift by pushing the ground away with your feet, driving your chest up, and extending your hips. Continue lifting until the sandbag rests in a vertical position on your lap.

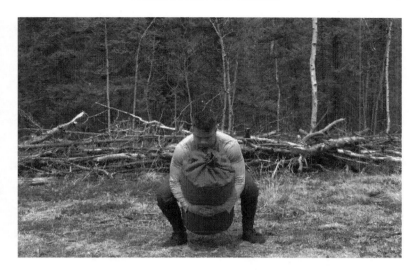

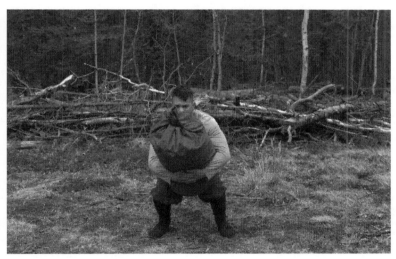

Variation 2: This variation is for extremely heavy sandbags. Wrap your arms around the sandbag with a bear hug grip, three quarters of the way up. Take a deep breath and brace, and squeeze the sandbag as hard as you can, hugging it to your chest. Lift by pushing the ground away with your feet, driving your chest up, and extending your hips. Once the sandbag is up

roughly halfway past your thighs, leverage it onto one leg by leaning it sideways. Reposition the sandbag as needed until it rests horizontally on your lap.

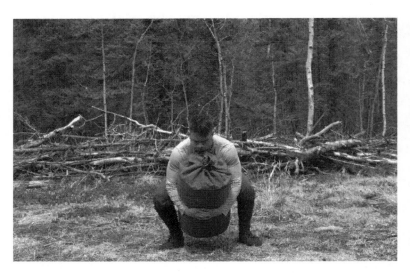

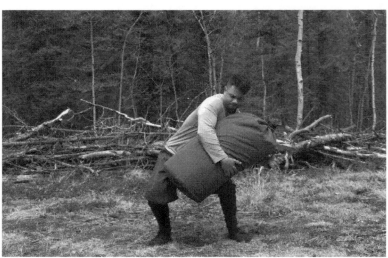

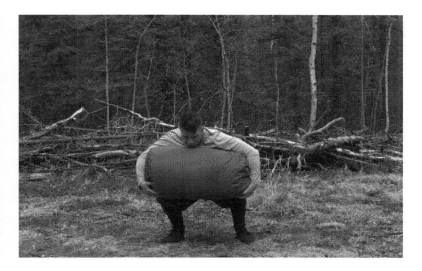

THE LIFT FROM THE GROUND: PROGRAMMING

The basic lift from the ground is very easy to program. Just follow these two principles:

1. Make sure at least 80% of the work you do with a sandbag starts from the ground.

If you plan on doing ten sets with a sandbag in a given session, at least eight of those sets should begin with you lifting the sandbag from the ground. You can't hope to improve your basic lifting strength if you don't train it directly, and a weak lift from the ground will eventually hold you back.

The temptation to start your sets by lifting the sandbag from a platform rather than from the ground will always be there, don't.

2. Always put everything you have into every lift.

It's easy to think of the lift from the ground as nothing more than an obstacle between you and other, more exciting movements. It's easy to imagine this part of lifting a sandbag wastes energy you could be using for other things, but this is looking at it in the wrong way. When done correctly, the lift from the ground will improve everything that follows.

Fast follows fast, slow follows slow.

If you view the lift from the ground as nothing more than a burden along the way you likely won't approach it with any kind of real intensity, and you'll end up lifting the sandbag slowly. A slow lift from the ground will make it much more difficult to reach the required level of intensity for whatever comes next.

If you attack that lift from the ground with everything you have, however, moving that sandbag as fast as you're able, the body will be primed and ready.

This concept is used by all the best strength athletes. A powerlifter knows every warm up set must be approached with a high level of effort. Powerful reps on the way to a max effort lift means a powerful max effort lift.

Using these two principals, you won't need to spend any part of your sandbag program doing sets dedicated entirely to the basic lift from the ground. Volume for this movement will be accumulated indirectly on the way to doing other things.

2

THE LIFT FROM THE LAP

THE LIFT from the lap is the most important movement in all of sandbag lifting. This position has a LOT of potential, and will determine your success with everything else moving forward.

If you want to carry a sandbag, bringing it higher up on your chest will help you to go much further.

If you want to throw a sandbag onto your shoulder, lifting it higher from the lap means less work later on when you're in a less advantageous position.

If you want to press a sandbag you first need to get it to the front rack position, which again means you must be strong from the lap.

To further understand the importance of the movement, let's compare it to a basic vertical jump, as jumping is actually very similar to lifting a sandbag. If your goal is to jump as high as you can, you'll instinctively initiate the jump by first crouching down, loading your body with tension like a spring. That tension is then used to propel you upwards. The most powerful jump happens when you're able to crouch down freely, bending at the ankles, knees, and hips. The subsequent extension of those three joints as you jump is known as 'triple extension'.

When a sandbag is resting on your lap, you're able to maximally load all three of those power producing joints. When you're standing upright with a sandbag held against your chest however, you lose the ability to create maximum tension in the hips. Power is generated by the knees and ankles alone, which will never be as powerful as true triple extension. Imagine trying to jump without bending your hips, it wouldn't work nearly as well.

When lifting a sandbag from the lap there are two main starting positions: vertical and horizontal. Each has its place, and every lifter will have their own preferences for how and when to use one or the other. One person might find a vertical lift lets them go much further during a carry, but a horizontal lift makes it easier to shoulder a sandbag. Others may find the opposite is true.

One lifter may prefer to ignore the horizontal lift altogether, another the vertical lift. It's up to you to decide which you prefer and when you prefer it.

Note: *How you lift a sandbag from the lap isn't necessarily determined by how you lift it from the ground. You can always reposition a sandbag as needed once it's on your lap.*

THE VERTICAL LIFT FROM THE LAP: HOW TO

There are two distinct methods you can use to lift a sandbag from your lap in a vertical position. One relies more on pure strength, while the other uses power and momentum. Both are used at the elite level, and both are viable long term. In either case, your goal should always be lifting the sandbag as high on your chest as you can.

Method 1:

The first lifting style relies on raw strength to get the job done. It's often slower moving and may feel more difficult at the start, but if you're able to pull it off it will land you in a good place.

Preparation is the most important part of this technique. Squat down low, grab low on the sandbag with a bear hug grip, and wedge your chest against the sandbag near its base. Once you're set, take a deep breath and brace, and stand up. Because you grabbed low down on the sandbag it should now be resting high up on your chest.

Method 2:

The second lifting style is focused on power and momentum. This method makes the initial lift from the lap easier but requires more skill to complete. To perform the movement, wrap your arms around the sandbag with a bear hug grip, some-where near the middle. This starting position will feel more comfortable as you won't need to squat down nearly as far. Take a deep breath and brace, and initiate the lift in the same way you would a vertical jump by pushing your hips backward, making your body like a spring.

Next, quickly reverse that movement by extending forward as explosively as you can, imagining as you do that you're trying to throw the sandbag up and over your head. As you hit max speed and reach an upright standing position, release your grip on the sandbag slightly, allowing it to continue moving upwards on its own. Once it's as high as it will go, catch it against your chest.

Where Method 1 was more like a squat, Method 2 is more like a throw.

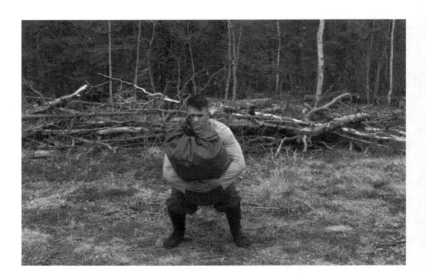

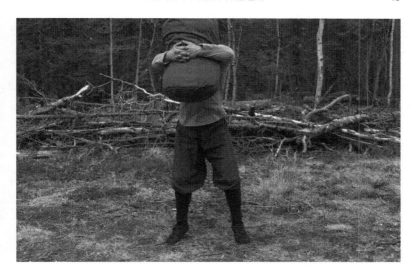

THE HORIZONTAL LIFT FROM THE LAP

The vertical lift from the lap is always very straightforward. Whether your goal is to lift a sandbag to chest height, to carry it, or to shoulder it, the sandbag always moves up in a straight line.

The horizontal lift has much more potential. Hand placement, the position of the sandbag on the lap, technique, and intention are all determined by what you plan on doing with the sandbag once you've lifted it. For now, let's assume your goal is standing upright with a sandbag and holding it there. There are two different techniques to choose from.

THE HIGH LIFT

From a vertical starting position, the lifting style was determined by how high or low you grabbed onto the sandbag. From a horizontal position, it's determined by how far around the sandbag you reach your arms. When attempting the high lift, your arms should be wrapped as far around the sandbag as you can get them. This makes the initial lift more difficult but will land the sandbag in a higher place on the chest.

THE HIGH LIFT: HOW TO

To perform the movement, squat down low and wrap your arms as far as you can either over top of the sandbag, or around the outsides. Take a deep breath and brace, and stand up, holding the sandbag tight against your body as you do. The sandbag should end high on your upper chest.

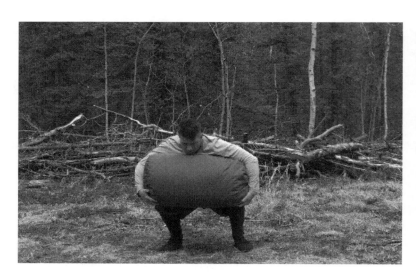

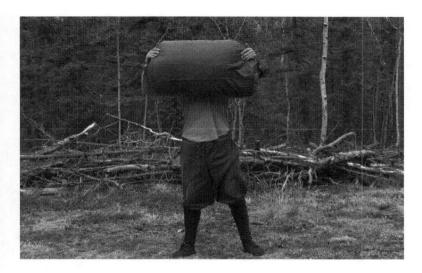

THE LOW LIFT

The low lift can be thought of as a partial version of the high lift. This may sound counterintuitive, but there are situations where this technique makes more sense. If you're not yet strong enough to bring a sandbag all the way to your upper chest, this variation can act as a stepping stone on your way there.

This lifting style can also be used to conserve energy. If you're in a race to move multiple sandbags over a short distance, for example, the low lift might help. The goal of this method is to stand completely upright while moving the sandbag only as much as is needed.

THE LOW LIFT: HOW TO

To perform the movement, reach your hands overtop of the sandbag, just far enough to keep hold of it. Take a deep breath and brace, and stand up. The sandbag should remain at or around waist level. In this position your hold on the sandbag won't be as strong, as you'll be relying more on friction than the strength of your muscles, but it will be enough for a short time.

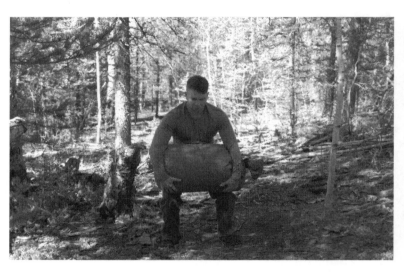

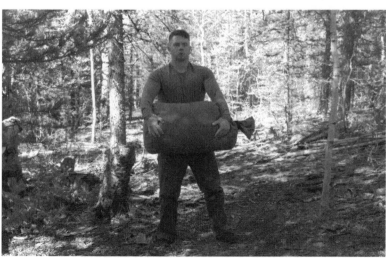

THE LIFT FROM THE LAP

THE LIFT FROM THE LAP: PROGRAMMING

The lift from the lap is a foundational exercise, it's something you need to do on your way to doing other things, which makes it very easy to program. Like the lift from the ground, most of the work for this exercise will be accumulated indirectly while doing other things. Unlike the lift from the ground however, spending some time focusing on the basic lift from the lap directly, as a standalone exercise is recommended.

Where you place this direct work in a training session will be determined by which lifting style you use. Both of the horizontal lifting methods, as well as vertical lifting Method 1 are all considered strength based exercises, so they'll go in the second 'strength based' half of a workout. Vertical lifting Method 2 has an element of power to it, so it works best in the first 'power-based' half of a workout.

The basic lift from the lap also requires far less mental willpower to perform at a high level than most other things, so it's best placed at the end of whichever section it's in.

A little goes a long way with these exercises. As stated before, you'll already be accumulating a lot of volume when working with other movements so you won't need much.

For vertical lifting Method 2, a basic 3-5 sets of 3 reps at the end of the power based section of a workout will be sufficient.

For the other strength-based lifting variations, one burnout set of max reps at the very end of a workout is effective.

3
THE SANDBAG CARRY

OF ALL THE exercises you can do with a sandbag, the carry is likely to have the greatest impact on your daily life. Traditional gym exercise can make you big and strong, but there's often something missing. There are often gaps in strength left behind that remain there indefinitely.

Sandbag carries fill in those gaps.

A heavy carry forces your entire body to work as one solid unit, and leaves you feeling stable on your feet in a way nothing else will. There's a confidence you get in the way you hold yourself, in your posture, and in the way you move. You develop a kind of certainty to your step that's hard to understand until you spend some time carrying heavy sandbags yourself.

There are many different carry variations, and they're all effective. When deciding which to choose, there are a few things to consider:

Purpose, Position (horizontal or vertical), and Height.

Purpose:

When deciding how to carry a sandbag, purpose should always be at the front of your mind.

What is it you hope to achieve with this carry?

Is the goal to move a sandbag from point A to point B as quickly as possible?

Will you eventually need to load the sandbag onto a platform, or can you drop it to the ground?

Is the carry meant as an accessory exercise for another movement, or are you just after the general strength, muscle, and conditioning benefits?

Knowing what your goals are beforehand will make any time spent carrying a sandbag much more impactful.

Position (Horizontal/Vertical):

Once you know why you're carrying the sandbag, it's time to decide on a position.

If your goal is to move as quickly as you can from point A to point B, choose whichever position you can get to in the least amount of time (this will likely depend on which style you prefer when lifting a sandbag from the ground).

If you need to load the sandbag onto a platform at the end of the carry, a horizontal position is probably best. Even if it initially takes you longer to get there, a horizontal position means more clearance under the bag and a higher likelihood you'll get it onto the platform.

If the carry is meant as an accessory exercise for another movement, bring the sandbag to the exact position you're trying to improve and keep it there.

If you're after the general benefits to strength, muscle, and conditioning, carry the sandbag in as many different positions as you can (horizontal, vertical, and every angle between the two).

Height:

Height also plays an important role in deciding where to hold a sandbag.

If you're after max speed over a short distance, holding the sandbag near waist level might save you some time. If you need to cover a large distance, holding the sandbag high up on your chest will be the better option (the higher you bring the sandbag, the more room it has to fall as your grip fatigues, and with a long distance carry you'll need every advantage you can get).

If your goal is becoming bigger and stronger in a general sense, a high carry position is more effective. When a sandbag is held high up on the body, all of the muscles below it have no choice but to work actively at all times to keep the body stable. When the sandbag is held lower down near waist level however, everything above it has a tendency to work only passively. More active work, over a larger area means better gains in strength and size.

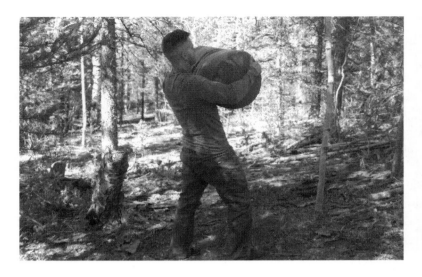

THE SANDBAG CARRY: HOW TO

The sandbag carry is simple and doesn't take long to master, but it's unforgiving and brutal. To perform the movement, combine everything from the previous chapters (lifting a sandbag from the ground to the lap, and from the lap to a standing position) and start walking. Here are a few tips to help you out:

Proud Chest/ Tall Spine

Try at all times to remain standing upright. Some backwards lean is inevitable as you fatigue, but your intention should be to keep a 'tall spine' and a 'proud chest'. This keeps the muscles engaged, and keeps tension where you want it.

Purposeful Steps

Every step you take should be intentional and uniform. Stride distance is up to personal preference, but do your best to make every step the same. Over time, mastering the way you walk with a sandbag will lead to improved speed, balance, and strength.

Breathing and Bracing

Breathing and bracing is the most difficult part to master when carrying a sandbag. It will be difficult when you first start, and it will continue being difficult years down the road.

With every step you take, the sandbag will fight you.

You must fight back.

With the sandbag resting on your lap, take in as much air as you can, and brace with everything you have, as if readying yourself for a punch to the gut. Maintain the brace as you stand up, and hold onto it as you walk. With every step, imagine your torso is unyielding, as if it's been cast from steel and no amount of pressure could cause it to collapse. As you walk, take quick, shallow breaths, letting each one reach all the way down to the pit of your stomach. Bit by bit, as time goes by the brace in your core will slowly give way to the pressure of the sandbag. It will happen, but you must fight for as long as you can.

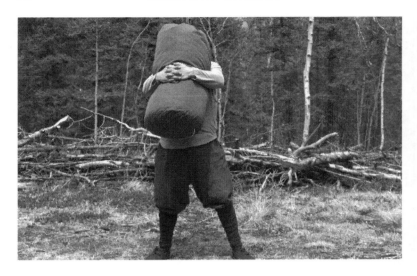

THE SANDBAG CARRY: MUSCLE

Stabilization

To better understand how the sandbag carry builds muscle, we need to go over stabilization. There are a lot of muscles in the human body. It's usually estimated there are at least 640 of them. Some are big, some are small. Some rarely act as stabilizers, and some almost always fill that role. Two things are certain:

1. When trained with intensity a muscle will grow, regardless of the role it plays (lifting, lowering, or stabilizing).
2. All muscles have the potential to stabilize the body.

At the base level, we can say a muscle is acting as a stabilizer when its purpose is preventing movement. When you do a barbell deadlift for example, the spinal erector muscles stabilize the spine and keep you from rounding forward. If however, you were to do something like a flexion row, where you actively flex and extend the spine, the spinal erectors would act as prime mover muscles.

Movers move, stabilizers stabilize.

A muscle can do both.

Looking again at the barbell deadlift, no one will tell you it's a bad exercise for growing and strengthening the spinal erectors. In fact, it's usually seen as one of the very best exercises for that purpose, even though there's no actual movement happening in those muscles.

Are the spinal erectors somehow special?

Do they for some reason adapt faster by stabilizing than other muscles do?

No.

Skeletal muscle is all made up of the same stuff. Viewed in isolation, apart from the body, spinal erector muscle would look identical to muscle from the upper arm. Fiber type distributions may be different between the two, but that doesn't change what they are.

If the spinal erectors grow very well by stabilizing, so too can every other muscle.

Enter the sandbag carry.

With the spinal erectors and the barbell deadlift as a guide, it should become clear why the sandbag carry builds so much muscle: stabilization.

When carrying a sandbag, the upper body remains rigid. There's no concentric, or eccentric lifting or lowering happening. Nearly every muscle from the waist up to the neck is tense and working to prevent movement.

The muscles of the torso work to keep the spine from bending.

The arms, chest, upper back and traps, as well as many other things all work isometrically to 'stabilize' the sandbag and keep it held in place.

That's when you're standing still.

When you start walking everything is magnified a thousand-fold. Every step you take sends a shock wave up the body which must be dampened, and controlled by the muscles.

This causes some pretty extreme adaptations.

Heavy Weight

Another thing to consider is the systemic effect of carrying a heavy sandbag. There seems to be something special about forcing the body to handle heavy weights that causes rapid gains in size and strength. You hear stories about this from every field of exercise.

The machine-focused gym goer starts doing heavy, free-weighted barbell squats and deadlifts and blows up in size. He finds that not only have the muscles associated directly with those exercises improved, but so has everything else as well.

The bodyweight calisthenics athlete adds weighted pull-ups to his routine and ends up looking like an entirely different person a few months later.

Do these things happen because those specific exercises are so effective, or is there more going on than first meets the eye?

Could it be loading the body with heavy weight in a general sense is what's responsible for the sudden improvements?

Our bodies are intelligent, and they want stasis. Survival is number one, and adapting to threats is something we're very good at. Loading the body with heavy weight is such a threat, and becoming bigger and stronger is the adaptation.

There are many different exercises you can use for this purpose, but nothing comes close to the sandbag carry.

If you take only one thing away from this entire book, let it be this: If your goal is becoming bigger and stronger, add some weighted carries to your program!

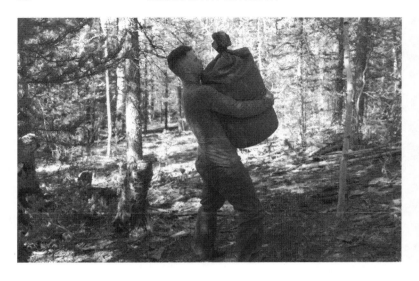

THE SANDBAG CARRY: PROGRAMMING

The lifts from the ground and from the lap usually act as stepping stones on the way to other things. Much of the work for those movements is accumulated indirectly as a result. The sandbag carry is a final destination, which makes programming it a bit more specific.

Considering again that a sandbag training day is made up of two distinct parts, power and strength, the sandbag carry is best placed at the beginning of the strength section of a workout.

This is for two reasons:

1. The sandbag carry is a strength-based exercise with a low skill requirement, and won't benefit much from the added power output you have at the start of a

workout. Placing the sandbag carry too early would be a waste of that power.

2. It's placed at the beginning of the strength section of a workout because it requires a high level of mental focus to do well. More than anything, the sandbag carry is a test of willpower. If you have the will, you can keep pushing for much longer than you might expect. If your mind is already worn out however, you won't make it nearly as far.

For these reasons, placement of the sandbag carry is very important. There's a fine line between when you start slowing down physically, and when mental focus begins to fade. The carry lives in the space between those two things.

Here are two examples of how you might add the sandbag carry to a training day:

Example One:

In example one, our lifter (we'll call him J) is focused primarily on mastering the sandbag-to-shoulder with a sandbag he only recently shouldered for the first time. The sandbag is becoming more manageable and he can successfully complete the lift 9 times out of 10, but it still takes every ounce of effort he has to do it.

The power phase of his workout will be spent shouldering relatively light sandbags for the practice and to accumulate volume, as well as shouldering the heavy sandbag 2-3 times per shoulder.

Once J begins slowing down, the power phase of his workout will be over. Physically he will feel some fatigue, but his mind will still be sharp as he's worked with only one exercise at this point.

This is the perfect place for the sandbag carry, so that's what he does next.

After 3 sets of max distance bear hug carries, J's mind and body will both be nearing their limits, but some strength will remain, enough to push one final time.

The only meaningful exercise worth doing at this point will be purely strength-based, and have a relatively small range of motion, preferably with space for rest between reps. With this in mind, J does one all-out set of max reps lifting a light sandbag from his lap in a vertical position and calls it a day.

Example Two:

In example two, J's goal is building strength with a newer, heavier sandbag from the ground to his lap, and from his lap to chest height, so he might one day become strong enough to shoulder it.

Technical and power-based movements need to come first in the workout, so first, to continue building power and skill with the movement, J shoulders a light sandbag 5-10 times per side before moving on to the heavy sandbag.

With the heavy sandbag he does three max intensity attempts lifting it from the ground to his lap, then up from his lap to chest height.

At the end of the final attempt, he places the heavy sandbag onto an elevated surface. From this elevated surface J does five singles, rolling the sandbag onto his lap and lifting it to chest height (this is done because the lift from the lap to chest height is much less fatiguing than the lift from the ground to the lap).

At this point, due to all of the extra strength work with the heavy sandbag, both J's body and mind will be exhausted and any attempts at carrying a sandbag would be unproductive, so he moves on.

To complete the workout J attempts one final set of max reps, lifting a light sandbag from his lap in a horizontal position and ends the workout.

With these examples you can see that where and when to place the sandbag carry in a workout is determined by your current goals.

4

THE SANDBAG-TO-SHOULDER

IF YOU'RE LOOKING for a reason to lift sandbags, this is it. The sandbag-to-shoulder is likely to be THE thing that keeps you coming back. Not only does it build tremendous total body strength and power, but the sandbag-to-shoulder is a lot of fun. So fun, in fact, there's an entire community of people out there centered around the sport that is shouldering heavy things. From stones, to pieces of scrap metal, if it can be lifted you can bet there's someone out there who's shouldered it. Sandbags are consistent, reliable, and straight to the point, which makes them a great place to start along this path.

At first glance, the sandbag-to-shoulder might seem like a straightforward exercise. Simply move a sandbag from point A to point B and you're done. From far away this might be true, but looked at more closely it becomes clear there's much more going on than that. There's much more to doing a thing than just getting it done. How you do it is just as meaningful, and with the sandbag-to-shoulder, the room for experimentation between points A and B is vast. The real joy of shouldering a heavy sandbag is in solving the puzzle that exists between those two points.

Every person is built differently, with different limb lengths and body shapes, strengths, weaknesses, and preferences, and given enough time each person will create a lifting style that is uniquely their own. All techniques are valid, there's no one particular lifting style used by everyone at the elite level, which means it's up to you to decide which you like best.

When the goal is shouldering the most amount of weight, you will inevitably find one method that suits you better than any other, but always remember there is strength to be gained from spending time with each variation of the movement.

VERTICAL

The most basic and straightforward way to shoulder a sandbag is from a vertical position on the lap. This lifting style relies entirely on the strength and power of the lifter, rather than the use of any special techniques. To better understand why this is, we need to compare it with its horizontal counterpart.

When shouldering a sandbag, regardless of where it starts or how it gets there, it will always need to end in a vertical position on the shoulder, it's the only way to maintain balance. This means when you start with a sandbag resting horizontally on your lap, at some point along the way it will need to rotate to an upright position.

This may lead you to believe a horizontal lift is unnecessary and only complicates the process, making things more difficult for the lifter, but this couldn't be further from the truth. Taking advantage of rotation on the way up to the shoulder can actually make things much easier. There is more skill involved in doing things this way, but the lifter who becomes a master with any of the more technical horizontal lifting variations will unlock the ability to shoulder weights they wouldn't otherwise have been able to when relying on raw strength alone.

The vertical lifting method isn't like this. There are no tricks or special techniques to rely on. When attempting to move a sandbag from the lap to the shoulder from a vertical starting position, you either have the strength to do it, or you don't. This makes it a great base builder for anyone starting out, as well as a great accessory exercise for anyone who prefers a horizontal lifting style.

VERTICAL: HOW TO

To perform the movement, start with a sandbag resting on your lap in a vertical position, and wrap your arms around it with a bear hug grip. Where you hold onto the sandbag will depend on your preferred lifting style (as discussed earlier in the chapter on the lift from the lap).

Take a deep breath and brace, and drive the sandbag up towards one shoulder. With a light sandbag, you may bring it all the way up in one powerful motion. If the sandbag is heavier, it may take you many heaves to reach the shoulder. Either way, always be sure to maintain a solid brace in your core.

It will help to imagine that with every push your intention is to throw the sandbag up and over your shoulder. Like the martial artist who breaks a board by punching through it, striking a point beyond the board itself, so too must your intention be to throw the sandbag further than is actually necessary.

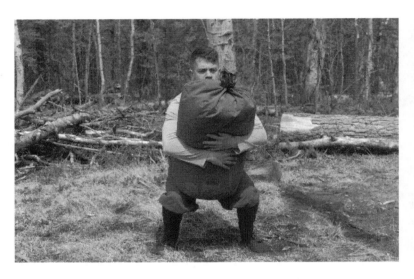

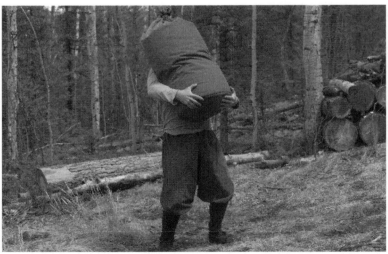

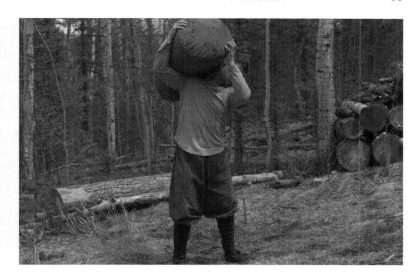

HORIZONTAL

Unlike the vertical lifting method which is very straightforward and has only the one variation, shouldering a sandbag from a horizontal position can be done a number of different ways depending on grip placement, and the degree of rotation used. The following lifting variations may have only minor differences between them, but sometimes one small adjustment can mean the difference between successfully shouldering a sandbag, and not. Once you've spent some time familiarizing yourself with the vertical lifting technique, it's recommended you work with both the following variations until you have a solid understanding of each.

One:

This lifting technique is a great next step when moving from the vertical lifting method to more technical variations, as it gets you comfortable lifting with an underhand grip in a safe and repeatable way. Your main focus when starting out with this technique should be on keeping your underhand arm rigid. You're lifting with your hips, not with your arms. Keep this in mind at all times.

To perform the movement, rest a sandbag horizontally on your lap with one arm over top, and one arm underneath. You may need to place the sandbag slightly off center, more towards the underhand side if it's not very long so you have space to wrap your arm underneath it. Take a deep breath and brace, and use your hips to drive the sandbag upwards. As you do this, use your underhand arm as a guide to flip the sandbag upright, either towards the shoulder on the same side as your underhand arm, or towards the opposite shoulder. Once the sandbag is in a vertical position on your chest, continue driving upwards with as many heaves as is necessary to complete the lift.

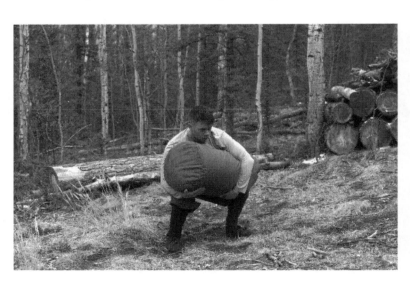

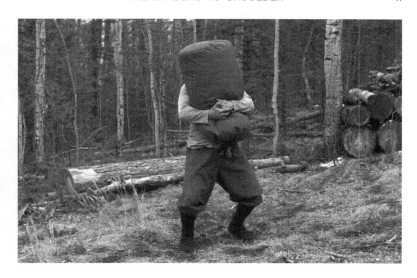

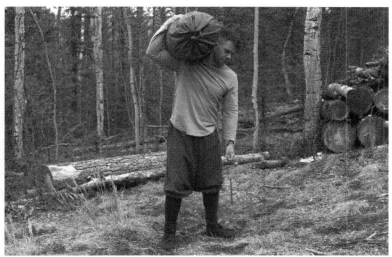

Two:

This lifting technique has a higher skill requirement and will take a great deal of practice to master, but once you have it down you'll find it puts you at a mechanical advantage during multiple parts of the lift.

To perform the movement, rest a sandbag horizontally on your lap and wrap both arms over top. This is a very powerful position to be in, and will give you an advantage from the start. Take a deep breath and brace, and drive the sandbag upwards, imagining your goal is to throw it up and over your head.

This is a power based technique, and your main focus should be on bringing the sandbag as high as you can with that first lift from the lap.

Once the sandbag is high up on your chest, reach one arm underneath and catch it. Your arms should now be in an over-under position. From here, as with the previous technique, use the underhand arm as a guide to flip the sandbag towards either the shoulder on the same side as the underhand arm, or to the opposite shoulder. There is a lot of timing and precision required with this technique, but once you master it you may just surprise yourself with what you're capable of.

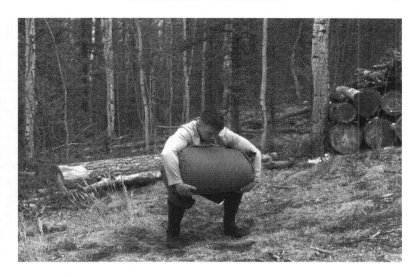

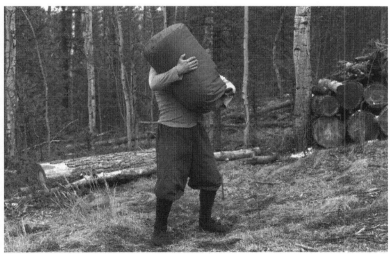

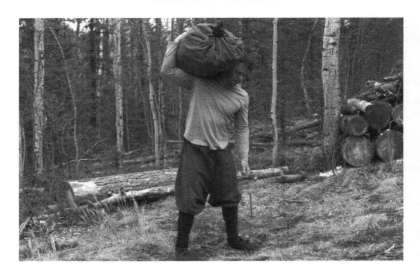

VARIATION

Mastering these horizontal lifting techniques will teach you the basics of grip position and rotation needed to shoulder a sandbag, but this is only the beginning. With a solid understanding of the fundamentals, it's time to experiment and search for your own unique lifting style. There is endless room for variation.

Which parts of the movement will you choose to focus on?

Are you strongest from the lap, or is it with a sandbag held at chest height you feel most powerful?

Do you prefer starting with an over-under grip, or do you like switching grips part way through?

Is the added power you get from a double overhand starting position worth the extra work you'll need to do later on?

Maybe you'll delay switching grips until the very end, or maybe you'll add an extra step somewhere in the middle.

As you become stronger and develop a real understanding of how a sandbag moves from one place to another, your preferred lifting style will become something that is uniquely yours.

The sandbag-to-shoulder technique that suits you best may not be obvious from the start, but given time you will find one that feels right.

Some prefer the simplicity of the vertical lifting method.

Others may prefer the most technical horizontal variations.

In the end, it all comes down to you as an individual.

Once you've found your technique, practice it as often as you can. Becoming a technical master with your preferred lifting style is a goal worth working towards, and the pursuit of that goal will change you.

BREATHING

Regardless of which technique you use to shoulder a sandbag, one thing is certain:

It will always be easier to take in a full breath of air when a sandbag rests on your lap, than it will be when it's pressing down on your chest.

This is a big deal because a solid brace is what keeps you safe from injury, and is often the determining factor in whether or not you successfully shoulder a sandbag.

This leaves you with two options:

1. You try to complete the entire lift quickly from the lap to the shoulder in one breath.
2. You accept a suboptimal brace and breathe along the way.

Actual sandbag-to-shoulder techniques aside, this is the most notable difference between lifters.

Here are a few tips for each.

SLOW AND CONTROLLED, BREATHING ALONG THE WAY

Breathing and bracing with a sandbag held against your chest will never be easy, but there are a few things you can do to make it easier. The first is to consider that every position is different. Breathing with a sandbag halfway to the shoulder is different from breathing when it's three quarters of the way there. Every different position is like a new skill that needs refining. The best way to develop those skills is with static holds, and carries.

If you want to improve at a specific point on the way to the shoulder, bring a sandbag to that position and keep it there for time, doing everything you can to hold onto your brace while breathing. This will be uncomfortable at first, but the results are worth the struggle.

You can set aside a few minutes of your workout to focus on this directly if you'd like, or you can use carries for some indirect work. If you already have 3 sets of sandbag carries programmed for a given training day, just do them with the sandbag held at whichever spot you need to work on and adjust that position over time as you improve.

ONE BREATH

Lifting a sandbag all the way from the lap to the shoulder in one breath is a trade off. You'll have more strength and power to complete the lift, but less time to do it. This means you'll need a very high level of skill if you want to pull it off. You'll need to know at an instinctual level where a sandbag will end up with each push, and what it takes to get there. Every step of the way from the lap to the shoulder needs to be intentional and precise. Hand placement, the amount of rotation needed, and every other little thing must become second nature.

For all of these reasons, the best way to improve the 'one breath' lifting style is to practice. Practice your technique over and over until it's perfect, then practice some more. Once you feel you're nearing perfect, keep going. If you want to lift this way, it's likely a very large portion of your time with a sandbag will be spent on the sandbag-to-shoulder. It takes a lot of dedicated work to maintain a high level of technical mastery, but it's worth it. A perfect shoulder attempt is a wonder to behold, and is worth every ounce of effort it takes to get there.

For some this is a discouraging thought, knowing there's so much work to do. For others, it's what makes the sandbag-to-shoulder such an enjoyable sport. Knowing the road to shouldering heavy things is long and full of obstacles, but that there is in fact a road to getting better can be a very motivating thought. Stumbling around in the dark is one thing, but with a clear-cut path in front of you, all it takes is another step.

Note on breathing: There is a big difference between holding your breath and doing something in one breath. HOLDING your breath can lead to lightheadedness, and in some extreme circumstances, passing out. The best way to avoid this is to make a quick 'tss' sound every time the sandbag lands in a new position.

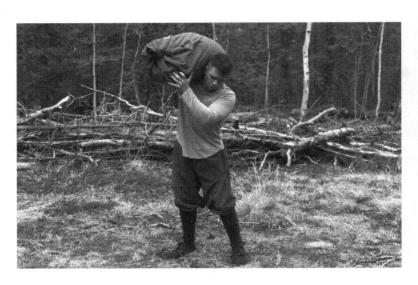

THE SANDBAG-TO-SHOULDER: THE DRIVING FORCE

In many ways, the sandbag-to-shoulder is the ultimate muscle-building exercise, but in many others, you could say it's nothing more than the sum of its parts. The three basic sandbag exercises discussed in previous chapters (the lift from the ground, from the lap, and the carry) work the body in almost the same way the sandbag-to-shoulder does. If you wanted, you could build a similar amount of muscle just by focusing on those three exercises and forget about shouldering heavy things altogether, but in doing so you'd be giving up something far greater.

Muscle, strength, power and the rest aside, the sandbag-to-shoulder gives you something much more significant: purpose.

Above all else, shouldering a sandbag is fun. It's less exercise and more game or sport, and if you plan on training for the rest of your life that's likely to be much more meaningful than anything else.

The moment you first manage to shoulder something heavy, you'll feel it.

A sudden shift in understanding.

"What have I been doing all this time?"

It's the realization that general physical abilities are nothing but a pale shadow on the ground when faced with the ever-burning sun that is learning a skill.

Learning to actually do something.

To use your body for a meaningful purpose.

In that moment of triumph, sandbag on your shoulder, the victor of this small battle, exercise takes on new meaning. No longer is the gym just a place you go to for all the normal reasons.

Every single thing you do from this point onwards will be in service of the sandbag-to-shoulder.

Muscle and strength?

Those things will come, there's no doubt about that. Every bit of weight you add to that sandbag will mean more size and strength, but you probably won't notice it.

Not at first.

Too much of your attention will be focused on performance above all else.

This is the true secret of the sandbag-to-shoulder. By not even thinking about muscle, you'll end up with much more of it.

An obsession with perfecting your skill means you become more consistent. You never miss a day in the gym. In fact, it becomes difficult to stay away.

Rather than, "What's the least amount of work I can do in the gym to become big and strong," your thoughts become, "How much can I get away with before I do too much?"

You see the same thing in other lifting sports.

The average muscle-driven gym person turned powerlifter becomes so obsessed with improving their squat, bench, and deadlift, that they wake up one day and realize they finally look like someone who lifts weights.

The calisthenics athlete becomes hyper-focused on mastering the planche, and when they finally achieve it their body has transformed into something new.

The track and field competitor becomes so hooked on improving power for the shot put, by the end of an off-season they realize their muscular development is on par with that of a bodybuilder.

This is why the sandbag-to-shoulder is the ultimate muscle-building exercise.

This is what makes all sandbag lifting so powerful.

It transforms you from just another person who goes to the gym to an athlete, and as an athlete, it's your job to play, and playing is never work.

It also just so happens that the sandbag-to-shoulder is a lifting sport with progressive overload in its bones, which means your reward for playing is becoming big and strong.

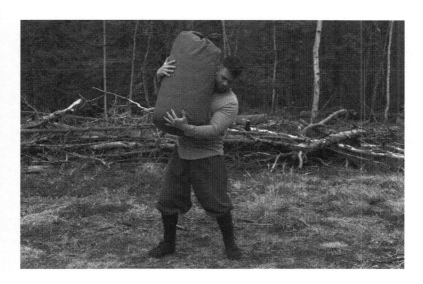

THE SANDBAG-TO-SHOULDER: UNLIMITED POWER

Have you ever had a dream where you're being chased, and you try to run away as fast as you can, but for some reason your body moves in slow motion? You try with everything you have to move just a LITTLE faster, but nothing seems to work. Your legs have become leaden, and there's nothing you can do.

This feeling happens more often than you might expect in the waking world when pushing the limits of high-intensity exercise. The body is strong and ready, the adrenaline says, "You've got this!" but somewhere beneath it all is a part of the mind that just won't have it. Like in the dream, you know you should have the strength to do what needs doing, but you can't seem to tap into it, so it feels like you're moving in slow motion.

Something about the heavy sandbag-to-shoulder, above all other things, has a direct line into this feeling.

Maybe it's the awkward, bulky nature of a sandbag or the feeling that you can't get a solid grip on the thing no matter how hard you try.

Maybe it's the hidden truth that the sandbag weighs more than a full-grown person, or the knowledge that you're actually planning on tossing that overgrown human-sized thing up onto your shoulder where it has a very real chance of folding you in half.

Maybe it's a bit of everything, but something about the sandbag-to-shoulder causes that 'moving in slow motion' response.

Dreams are one thing, but when you're awake you can always do something. Just as with any other skill, the ability to push past that mental barrier can be trained. The ability to reach your true strength potential is something you can work towards with time.

The reason the sandbag-to-shoulder works so well for this is because you can't fake it. No half effort will be tolerated. To shoulder anything even remotely heavy, you will need 100% max effort intensity from start to finish. From the moment that sandbag leaves the ground, all the way until it reaches your shoulder, you'll need continuous and unyielding, life or death-like drive.

Eventually you'll reach a point where your body surpasses your mind. You'll be working towards a new, heavier sandbag, and you'll know the strength is there, but your mind won't yet allow it.

This is the turning point, the point in your training that will decide whether you have what it takes to become truly strong, or if you'll stay less than that forever.

You must keep pushing.

Keep shouldering sandbags that require 100% effort week after week, month after month. Keep at it and one day you'll notice a shift, as if all this time your mind has contained within it a well of power that has, up until now, been frozen solid. With every sandbag-to-shoulder attempt you've been chipping away at the ice, and finally, seemingly all at once, you've broken through.

This is what sandbag-to-shoulder specialization can do for you. It's the waking world equivalent to finding yourself in that slow-motion dream and suddenly gaining the ability to jump high into the sky and fly around the earth, far away from whatever scary thing was chasing you.

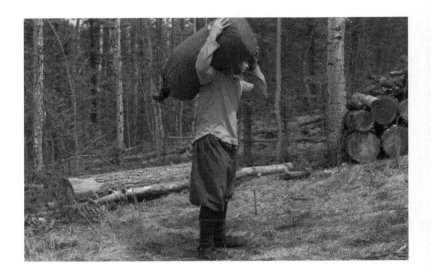

THE SANDBAG-TO-SHOULDER: PROGRAMMING

The sandbag-to-shoulder is best developed as a skill rather than as just another exercise. Every attempt must be done from a state of complete readiness, and technical mastery should always be at the front of your mind. Nothing should be allowed to come between you and the perfect rep, not temporary muscular fatigue, not being out of breath, nothing.

For these reasons, when working with the sandbag-to-shoulder, singles are best. Perfect practice makes records, and your technique will not be perfect when doing sets of 10. With high-rep sets, the body will try to compensate for muscular fatigue in ways you don't want, which can lead to bad habits. That's not to say you need ten minutes rest between every rep, that would take too long, but giving yourself enough time between reps so that each one starts from a place of true power will lead to far better long-term results.

You see a similar approach in Olympic Weightlifting. Rarely if ever will an Olympic weightlifter do more than 1-3 reps in a set when working with the full snatch, or clean and jerk. With accessory exercises, of course, sets of 10 and beyond are great, but never with the competition movements.

The total number of reps you'll do in a workout will require some self-awareness. The sandbag-to-shoulder takes a lot out of you quickly, and continuing on when you're already in a highly fatigued state is counterproductive. You'll want to stop doing the exercise for the day once your technique starts to break down, or when you start failing attempts. Typically this will be somewhere between 5 to 15 reps per shoulder (10 to 30 total attempts). If you can manage more than 15 reps per side in a single workout, it's likely time to move on to a heavier sandbag. If you can't do at least 5, you may wish to spend more time with lighter sandbags to accumulate volume, and to practice your technique.

This may seem like a low-volume approach, especially if your goal is building muscle with the movement, but over time the reps add up. A program focused on the sandbag-to-shoulder will typically have you training with a higher frequency, so while daily volume may be relatively low, monthly volume remains high. Even at the very lowest end, 5 reps per shoulder done twice a week is still 40 high-quality reps per shoulder every month.

Also, remember this only applies to the full ground-to-shoulder lift, you will accumulate much more total volume when factoring in other sandbag exercises as well.

Programming the sandbag-to-shoulder is very straightforward. It's a power-based movement, and will likely be the most technical exercise in a sandbag training routine, therefore it will almost always go first in a workout. Simply warm up, do as many perfect reps as you're able before fatigue sets in, and move on.

CHALLENGE SANDBAGS

If you're currently working towards shouldering a new, heavier sandbag, give yourself three attempts once per week to do it. If you successfully complete the lift on your first attempt, stop there and move on to whatever comes next (this could be more work shouldering lighter sandbags, or it could be moving on to another exercise). Do the same if you fail all three attempts.

The temptation to do more will always be there, but that would only set you back. Too much time spent trying, and failing to shoulder a max effort sandbag will quickly lead to excessive central nervous system fatigue, which means at best you'll need to deload sooner, and worst case scenario you'll end up hurting yourself.

Whether you're able to successfully lift your current challenge sandbag or not, the majority of your time should always be spent with relatively lighter sandbags, perfecting your technique and accumulating volume.

When working with a new sandbag it's best to use a slow and methodical approach.

If you successfully shoulder a sandbag in week one, wait until week two to try again.

If you successfully shoulder the sandbag again in week two, you can slowly begin adding volume.

In week three try for a single successful attempt on two different days.

If you manage that, do the same again in week four.

If that's successful, try for three attempts in week five, and so on.

In this way you'll slowly adjust to the heavier weight, eventually changing it from a challenge sandbag to a sandbag you could shoulder on any given day.

5
THE PRESS

FOR MANY LIFTERS, the sandbag-to-shoulder is the end goal.

The final destination.

The final movement that represents complete mastery with a sandbag.

For many lifters, this is enough. But for a select few, one final test remains:

The sandbag press.

The press represents a shift into new territory when compared with the other movements outlined thus far. The lift from the ground to the lap, from the lap to chest height, the carry, and the shoulder all exist in the same relative space. You might say each of these represents a different branch on a tree. Every branch is different, but they're all part of the same tree.

The press stems from entirely different roots.

As the name implies, the press involves the as yet largely neglected pressing muscles, those being the shoulders, triceps and chest mainly. While these muscles may have seen some minor involvement with the other posterior chain-based exercises, they acted mainly as support, functioning in the background.

With the press they're front and center.

Muscle isn't the only difference between movements however. The press is fundamentally different from other sandbag exercises in the way it makes your body work. With the four previous movements the sandbag always stayed close to the body's center, close to the torso. If you ever felt like you might lose control of the sandbag, you could always compensate by squeezing harder, or by pausing briefly mid-rep before continuing on.

When pressing a sandbag it's moved to a place that's as far away from the body's center as it can be. This requires an even greater level of breathing and bracing control and brings a new element of balance to the mix.

Because of these fundamental differences, you could be a master at the sandbag-to-shoulder, throwing heavy things weighing hundreds of pounds more than your own body weight up onto your shoulder, and still be a beginner at the press.

The path to pressing heavy sandbags is long and difficult, but for those few who can't resist the call, the feeling of unearthly power that comes with showing your complete dominion over a heavy awkward object is well worth the fight.

THE SANDBAG PRESS: HOW TO

The sandbag press is made up of two distinct parts:

The clean to the front rack position, and the press overhead.

The clean can be done using two different methods, one relying purely on raw strength, and the other making use of power and momentum to get the job done.

Method 1: Strength Clean

To perform the strength clean, rest a sandbag horizontally on your lap, squat down as low as you can, wedge yourself against the sandbag so your chin rests just above it, and wrap your arms around the outsides, as low as you can manage. Take a deep breath and brace, and lift straight up. The sandbag should now be held on the upper chest, close to your neck.

From here, change your hand position so your palms are underneath the sandbag, and your fingertips are facing up, wrapped around the outsides. You may need to lean back a bit to maintain your balance in this position, just be sure to lean at the hips rather than arching the lower back excessively.

Method 2: Power Clean

To perform the power clean, rest a sandbag horizontally on your lap and wrap your arms over top of it. Take a deep breath and brace, and drive the sandbag up with as much explosive power as you can manage. As the sandbag reaches neck and face level, 'catch' it in the front rack position, with your palms underneath, and your fingertips wrapped around the outsides.

In the front rack position your primary focus should be on making your body rigid to give yourself a solid base to press from. Keep your quads and glutes flexed at all times, imagining you're flexing them up towards your hips, while at the same time bracing your lats and core, imagining you're flexing them down towards your hips.

Quads and glutes up.

Lats and core down.

Maintain this position at all times during the press.

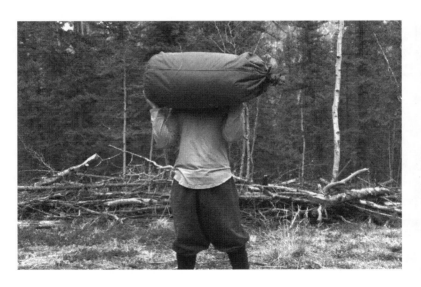

From here there are many different methods you can use to press the sandbag overhead. If you want to maximize your potential you can use techniques taken from the world of Olympic Weightlifting, using any number of different jerk variations. These can be very effective, but often require specialized coaching to get down properly. Discussing them in book format would be a massive undertaking so let's leave it at that for now. If you get hooked on the sandbag press, just know those weightlifting techniques are out there, and may be worth learning somewhere down the line.

Olympic variations aside, let's go over the two most basic pressing techniques: the strict press, and the push press.

STRICT PRESS

The strict press is a pure strength movement and relies solely on the strength of your pressing muscles. To perform the movement, simply press the sandbag overhead from the front rack position while keeping your knees locked out.

PUSH PRESS

The push press relies more on power and momentum, and often means heavier weights lifted. From the front rack position, quickly bend your knees, storing up energy, then reverse the motion as if you were going to jump. The force generated by your legs will transfer into the sandbag as you press it overhead.

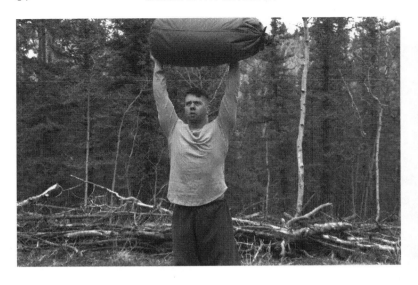

THE SANDBAG PRESS: PROGRAMMING

To truly master pressing a sandbag overhead, it will need to take priority in your program. You can't go in only halfway with this exercise. Unyielding dedication over many months and years is the only way forward. If elite pressing strength is your goal there will need to be some kind of compromise, and most likely that compromise will come in the form of the sandbag-to-shoulder. While you can work with both at the same time, they will interfere with each other. It'd be like playing two sports at once. Sure you can do it, and you can get pretty good at both, but you'll never become quite as advanced in either.

It may sound extreme, but you need to become just a bit obsessed with these movements if you want to master them. You need a level of dedication beyond just showing up to the gym.

Anyone who's reached a very high level with either of these movements will tell you the training doesn't stop when the workout ends. They're constantly thinking about their sport when moving through life, practicing the steps in their mind and imagining ways to improve.

They eat, sleep, and breathe this stuff.

In a general strength training context you can focus on both at the same time, just know if you want to be the absolute best in any one area, you'll need to specialize.

With that in mind, how you program the press depends on what your goals are. If you want to become the strongest presser ever, it will need to come first in your workouts, and you'll want to work with the movement at least twice a week, three times would be even better.

For the same reasons as with the sandbag-to-shoulder, when the aim is becoming as strong as humanly possible, singles are best. Working with singles lets you dial in your technique and ensures every rep is done with max strength and power. Anywhere from 5 to 15 heavy singles done at the start of a workout will serve you well.

If you're pushing towards a new, heavier sandbag, use the strategy outlined in the sandbag-to-shoulder section and give yourself three attempts once a week, and so on from there. After the heavy singles, drop down to a lighter sandbag and accumulate some volume with a basic 3 sets of 5-20 reps.

Note: When doing your heavy singles, start from the ground between every rep. When doing your rep work, there's no need to reset on the ground between reps.

If your goal is becoming as powerful as you can with both the sandbag-to-shoulder and the press at the same time, alternate which movement takes priority throughout the week. If you lift sandbags twice a week, day one will start with the heavy sandbag-to-shoulder, followed by the press for lighter weight sets of 5-20 reps. Day two will begin with heavy pressing work, followed by sandbag-to-shoulder practice with lighter sandbags, followed by lighter weight sets of 5-20 reps for the press.

Note: Getting stronger at the press requires more volume than the sandbag-to-shoulder does, so regardless of which movement took priority for the day, you'll always want to be sure to do your rep work for the press.

If your primary goal is the sandbag-to-shoulder, and the press is a secondary goal, place it first in the 'strength' section of your workouts. In this scenario, begin your workouts with the sandbag-to-shoulder, followed by any power-based accessory movements, then move on to pressing, and finish with carries, or whatever other strength-based movements you have planned for the day.

If you don't care about becoming a master of the sandbag press, but you still want the muscle building effects, place it last or near the end of your workouts, using higher rep sets.

6

THE ONE-MOTION SANDBAG-TO-SHOULDER

DRAWING on every bit of skill, power and strength developed with every other sandbag exercise discussed thus far, one final movement remains.

The ultimate display of total body strength and power.

The one-motion sandbag-to-shoulder.

This movement represents a division between those involved with shouldering heavy things. Talk with any number of lifters who have spent some time with it and you're likely to get one of two answers: either the one-motion sandbag-to-shoulder is the greatest movement of all time, or it's the worst. This mainly comes down to whether or not a lifter enjoys a challenge for the sake of itself, and whether or not they're willing to work with lighter weights.

When compared with traditional shouldering methods from the lap, the one-motion lift from the ground to the shoulder requires considerable skill and precision. For this reason, a big time investment is needed.

It's like mastering some form of jumping, spinning sidekick. Sure you could just do the reliable, ordinary sidekick and the end result would be relatively the same, but something about getting to that end place with a perfectly executed jump and spin is a wonder to see.

Love it or hate it, the one-motion sandbag-to-shoulder is an awesome display of mastery with a sandbag.

THE ONE-MOTION SANDBAG-TO-SHOULDER: HOW TO

The one-motion sandbag-to-shoulder is made up of two distinct parts:

The row, and the extension.

Begin with a sandbag horizontally on the ground and grab the outsides of it, palms facing towards each other. Take a deep breath and brace, and row the sandbag to your chest while maintaining a completely horizontal torso angle. Right as the sandbag reaches your chest, perform a 'good morning' movement by extending your hips and raising your chest. This hip extension will generate power, which will be transferred completely into the sandbag as you reach a fully upright standing position.

Using that power, imagine your goal is to throw the sandbag up and over your head, while at the same time rotating one side so it lands directly on the shoulder.

The entire process should be done in one fluid motion.

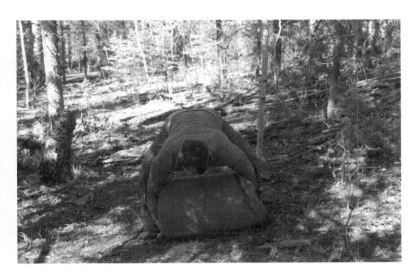

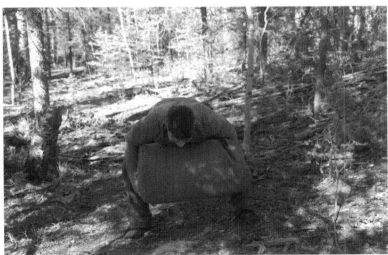

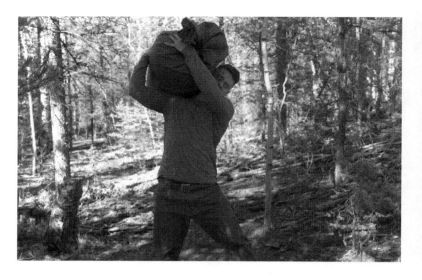

THE ONE-MOTION SANDBAG-TO-SHOULDER: PROGRAMMING

Mastering the one-motion sandbag-to-shoulder will require dedicated practice and every bit of power you have. It must become the primary focus of your workouts, and anything less than 100% effort will not work.

That said, it's still better to work with the standard sandbag-to-shoulder first in your workouts. This way you'll make sure you're properly warmed up, and that your standard technique doesn't deteriorate.

If the one-motion sandbag-to-shoulder is a priority, add it in place of the second half of your normal shouldering work. If your regularly scheduled workout calls for 10 shoulders per side in the normal way, instead do five the normal way, and five one-motions. A good strategy is to work up to shouldering your heaviest sandbag once per side, then move on to one-motion work.

An example training day might go as follows:

Ground-to-shoulder normal style:

200 lbs to each shoulder x2

225 lbs to each shoulder x1

250 lbs to each shoulder x1

One-Motion:

175 lbs to each shoulder x5

7
SANDBAG ACCESSORY MOVEMENTS

WITH A SOLID UNDERSTANDING of the five basic
fundamental sandbag exercises (the lift from the ground, the
lift from the lap, the carry, the shoulder, and the press) we can
move on to other, more situational movements. As nice as it
would be to continue indefinitely making linear progress on all
five of the basic exercises at the same time, strength doesn't
usually happen all at once. As you become stronger, some areas
will move ahead, while others fall behind. The goal with the
following accessory movements is to lessen that gap in strength.
These things act as tools that, when used strategically, ensure
no one thing holds back everything else.

Adding some variety to your program also goes a long way
towards keeping training enjoyable, and inevitably leads to a
more well-rounded physique.

Every second spent with a sandbag in your hands adds up, and
everything you do works synergistically with everything else.
Although the following exercises will be separated into cate-

gories based on what they help with most, keep in mind that just because an exercise is in one category doesn't mean it won't also help with another.

WEAK FROM THE GROUND:

The Sandbag Row

When working with sandbags it's easy to forget about leg drive. Most of what you do is posterior chain dominant, and the back and core are often prioritized above all else, while the legs become nothing more than an afterthought. Never is this more of a mistake than when lifting a sandbag from the ground. The legs are powerful, and using them correctly will allow you to lift much heavier weights. Sometimes all it takes to break through a perceived plateau is reminding yourself of that truth.

The sandbag row does this better than anything else. In addition to strengthening the body in the most awkward possible position, the row teaches leg drive and forces proper lifting mechanics.

There are many different techniques you can use to row a sandbag, but for our purposes here you'll want to mimic a barbell pendlay row.

THE SANDBAG ROW: HOW TO

To perform the movement, start with a sandbag resting horizontally on the ground and stand directly over top of it. Reach your hands underneath the outsides of the sandbag, palms facing towards each other. From this position, your torso angle should be parallel to the ground, and your knees should be slightly bent.

You must maintain this position at all times during the set.

Take a deep breath and brace, and row the sandbag to your chest by pushing the ground away with your feet and driving your elbows up. Once the sandbag reaches the top position, guide it back down to the ground with as much control as you can manage. Reset with the sandbag resting on the ground between every rep.

Note: If you're used to picking up a sandbag by 'lifting' rather than by 'pressing the ground away' it may take you a few sets to get a feel for it, but as you fatigue you'll have no choice but to do things correctly. This is part of why the sandbag row works so well for building leg drive. Because that bent-over position is so difficult to maintain, the body will do whatever it can to make the movement easier, and leg drive does just that.

THE SANDBAG ROW: PROGRAMMING

The sandbag row is a hybrid strength and power movement, and when used for the purpose of building strength off the ground, is best placed at the end of the power section of a workout.

Perfect practice with explosive intent should be the goal, therefore high sets and low reps works best. With low rep sets, every rep is done explosively, and the risk of injury is reduced substantially. Anywhere from 5 to 10 sets of 3 to 5 reps works well.

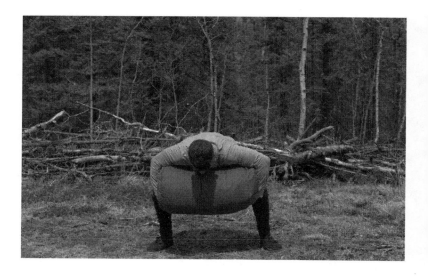

THE ONE-MOTION GROUND TO CHEST

Another reason strength off the ground falls behind is a lack of follow through. When moving a sandbag from the ground to the lap, the mind may begin slowing you down three quarters of the way up. This is because the end destination of the movement was set too low. When lifting a sandbag from the ground, the goal in your mind should actually be to lift it all the way up to your chest, not just to your lap. We can make sense of this using the barbell bench press as an example.

When pressing a barbell up from your chest, you begin with max power output at the bottom of the rep, but as you near lockout the body intuitively puts on the brakes so it doesn't fly out of your hands and come crashing down on you. If max power was maintained during the entire rep you would lose control of the barbell.

You cannot allow the body to think this way when lifting a sandbag.

Rather than a barbell bench press, you'll want to think in terms of its counter-movement, a medicine ball throw.

With a throw, max power is maintained at all times during the rep, which is exactly what you want with sandbags. It will benefit you greatly to imagine every part of sandbag lifting as a throw, always following through beyond the actual end destination.

One way to train this for a stronger lift from the ground is to lift a sandbag all the way from the ground to chest height in one-motion. There are two ways to do this depending on the position of the sandbag on the ground.

THE ONE-MOTION GROUND TO CHEST: HOW TO

Standing Upright

With a sandbag resting in an upright standing position on the ground, wrap your arms around it with a bear hug grip and lift straight up. Rather than stopping when you reach your lap, keep driving upwards until you're standing all the way up with the sandbag held against your chest.

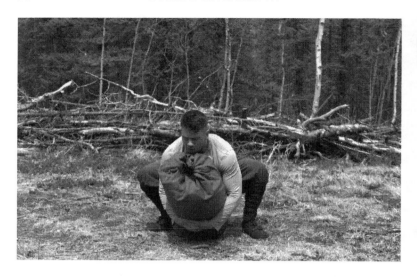

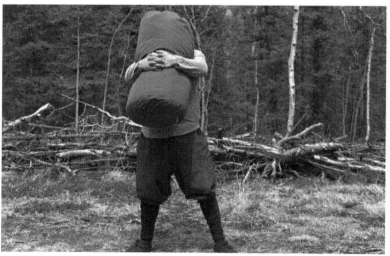

Horizontal

You can think of this exercise as being made up of two parts: a row, and a good morning. It's done in exactly the same way as the first part of a one-motion sandbag-to-shoulder, which also makes this a good accessory exercise for that.

With a sandbag resting horizontally on the ground, row it to your chest while maintaining a horizontal torso angle. Once there, perform a good morning (extend your hips and raise your chest until you're standing upright).

When first working with this movement, pause briefly between the two parts to build a solid understanding of each. Once you're familiar with each part, work on combining the two into one fluid movement, extending the hips and raising the chest right as the sandbag reaches chest height.

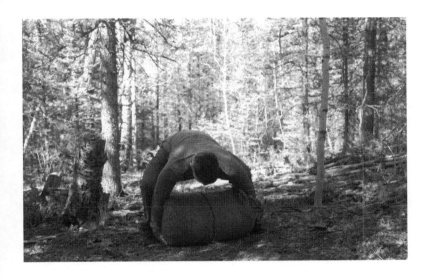

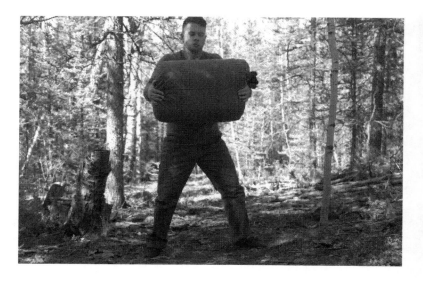

THE ONE-MOTION GROUND TO CHEST: PROGRAMMING

If the lift from the ground is truly a weak point, this is one of the few circumstances where an accessory exercise should go first in a workout, before the sandbag-to-shoulder or sandbag press. At the start of a workout, after you've warmed up, perform 3-5 singles with 1-2 minutes rest between reps lifting a sandbag from the ground to chest height in one-motion.

A little goes a long way with this exercise. Three to five quality reps will strengthen your weak point without taking too much away from the big, technical movements.

WEAK OFF THE LAP

If you want to master sandbag lifting, the lift from the lap must not become a weak point. In fact, it would be beneficial to do everything in your power to make it a strong point and keep it that way.

Similar to the section on improving strength from the ground, the best exercises for improving strength from the lap will focus on leg drive, and the follow-through.

THE SANDBAG SQUAT

The sandbag squat is to the lift from the lap what the row is to the lift from the ground. To perform the movement, hold a sandbag against your chest in a vertical position with a bear hug grip, and take a wide stance (you'll want your feet far enough apart so the sandbag has room to travel between your legs on the way down). Take a deep breath and brace, and squat down as low as is comfortable, somewhere near parallel. Once you reach the bottom position, squat back up by pushing the ground away with your feet, and driving your chest up.

Note: Holding the sandbag in a vertical position against the chest allows for a full range of motion, and makes the exercise much more useful for developing strength off the lap. With a sandbag held in a horizontal position, there's a tendency to cheat the movement by using the thighs for support at the bottom of every rep. This would take away from the added leg drive benefits we're after and makes the exercise much less effective.

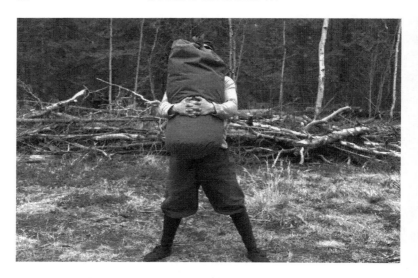

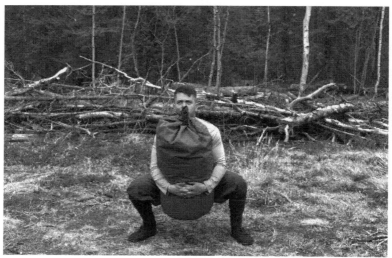

THE SANDBAG SQUAT: PROGRAMMING

The sandbag squat works best in the strength phase of a workout, directly after carries or in place of them. You can get away with doing higher rep sets of squats compared to most other things if your conditioning allows for it, so anything from three sets of ten reps, to ten sets of three reps can be effective.

THE SANDBAG BOX SQUAT

Breaking up the concentric and eccentric (lifting and lowering) parts of a squat by resting on a box at the bottom of every rep improves your ability to generate power from a deadstop, and makes the exercise more of a hybrid between a squat, and a basic lift from the lap to chest height. This makes the exercise very effective at teaching you to involve the legs more when lifting a sandbag from the lap.

THE BOX

Box height should be set low enough so you reach parallel or slightly above it at the bottom of the squat. This will generally be somewhere between 1-2 feet off the ground. A plyometric box or a bench both work well for this purpose. A sandbag can also be used.

THE SANDBAG BOX SQUAT: HOW TO

To perform the movement, hold a sandbag with either a vertical or horizontal grip, and squat down until you're resting on the box. Pause for at least 1-3 seconds in the bottom position to make sure all momentum has gone away, and stand back up.

Note: The movement is much more effective for building leg drive when done from a complete dead stop. Avoid the tempta-

tion to 'rock' yourself out of the bottom position by shifting your weight on the box.

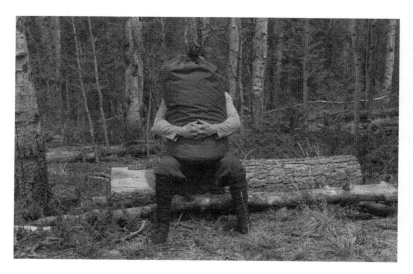

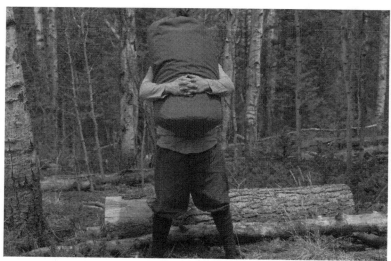

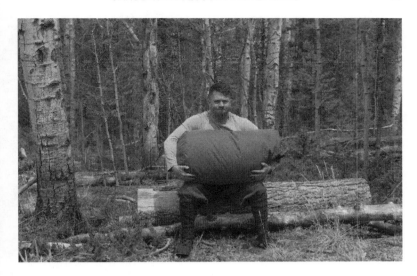

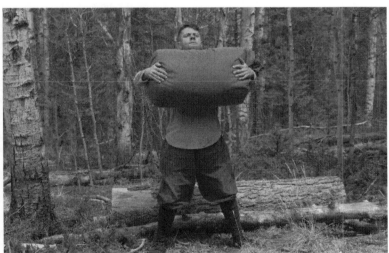

THE SANDBAG BOX SQUAT: PROGRAMMING

The sandbag box squat is a pure strength movement and works best near the end of the strength phase of a workout. Similar to the standard sandbag squat, the box squat can be done in most rep ranges.

The one major difference between the two is grip strength. With a standard squat you need to maintain a solid grip on the sandbag at all times, which means your grip might become the limiting factor. With a box squat, you're able to rest and regrip at the bottom of every rep, which lets you push the movement much further. For that reason, with the sandbag box squat, one all-out set of max reps also works well and makes for a great finisher to a workout.

THE SANDBAG HIGH PULL

If you shoulder a sandbag from a horizontal starting position on the lap, the sandbag high pull is likely to be the ultimate accessory exercise for you. This is a power movement through and through, and it will teach you to be much more explosive from the lap.

THE SANDBAG HIGH PULL: HOW TO

To get the most out of the sandbag high pull, it's best to think of it as a vertical jump with a sandbag held in your hands. To perform the movement, rest a sandbag horizontally on your lap and wrap both arms over top of it. Take a deep breath and brace, and initiate the movement by pushing your hips backwards, like you would when preparing for a jump, storing up energy like a spring ready to uncoil. From this place of complete power, explosively extend your hips, imagining as you do that your goal is to simultaneously jump into the air, and throw the sandbag over and behind your head. Once the sandbag reaches max height, let it drop back down to your lap and repeat for reps.

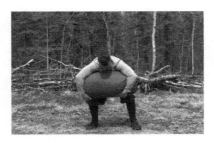

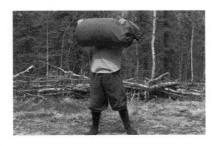

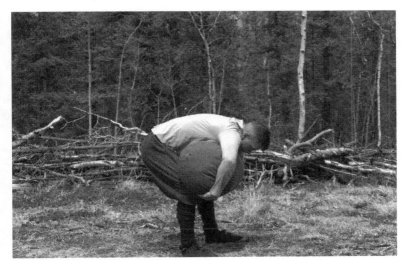

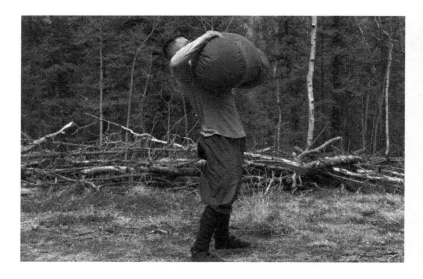

THE SANDBAG HIGH PULL: PROGRAMMING

In many ways the sandbag high pull is a deconstructed version of the full sandbag-to-shoulder. It lets you focus on the most important part of shouldering a sandbag without needing to worry about the rest of the movement. This makes it invaluable for lifters who rely on power above all else.

The high pull also lets you extend the max power section of a workout longer than would be possible if your only power based exercise was the full ground to shoulder lift. Once you've hit your daily limit for productive shoulder attempts, continuing on with the exercise is a bad idea. Your technique will suffer, and all you'll be doing is adding unnecessary fatigue for very little benefit.

Just because you've reached your limit for shouldering a sandbag though, doesn't mean you've reached the point where

ALL power movements become unproductive. Because the high pull is less technical, you can keep pushing at a high level of intensity for much longer than you ever could with the full sandbag-to-shoulder alone.

Depending on your energy level and the rest of the training day, perform anywhere from 5-10 sets of 3 reps with the sandbag high pull after your full sandbag-to-shoulder work. Move on to something else when you reach the point where you're no longer able to consistently lift the sandbag explosively.

SANDBAG LOADING

The other 'follow through' movement for the lift from the lap is sandbag loading. This should be thought of as exactly the same as the high pull, only with a tangible endpoint. The one downside to the high pull is accountability. Without a set end destination, it takes a great deal of self-awareness to accept when you're not lifting the sandbag as high as you should be. With a loading event there's no guesswork, either you make it or you don't.

There are plenty of different setups you can use for the exercise. An actual loading platform is ideal, but anything will do.

If your gym has a power rack, you can lift the sandbag up and over a barbell set on pins, and raise the pin height over time.

You can also loop a band around the pins, or use a sturdy 2x4 with the same result.

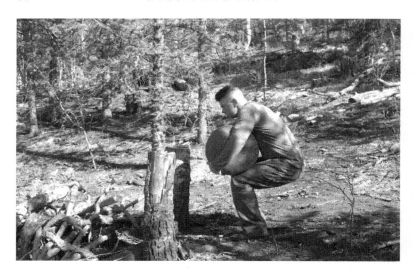

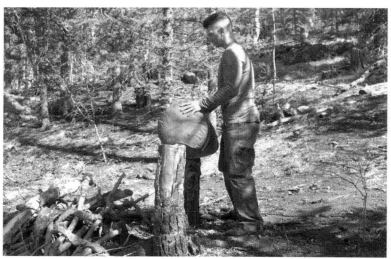

Sandbag loading requires some extra equipment, and possibly some extra creativity, but works very well for improving strength off the lap if you can figure it out. Program the exercise in the same way you would the high pull.

WEAK FROM CHEST HEIGHT TO SHOULDER

Difficulty completing the final part of a shoulder attempt (from the chest to the shoulder) usually comes down to one of two things:

A weak core, or a lack of skill.

Often the best way to improve these things is to spend more time practicing shouldering light sandbags, but there are a few specific things you can do to speed up the process.

THE SANDBAG SHOULDER CARRY

Shouldering a sandbag requires a type of core stability rarely developed with traditional training methods. With a sandbag held off-center, high up on your chest, more than anything you must fight to keep from falling to the side.

You can train this strength directly with the shoulder carry.

To perform the movement, lift a sandbag to one shoulder, hold onto it with both hands and start walking. Maintain a solid brace in your core at all times, and fight to stay as upright as you can.

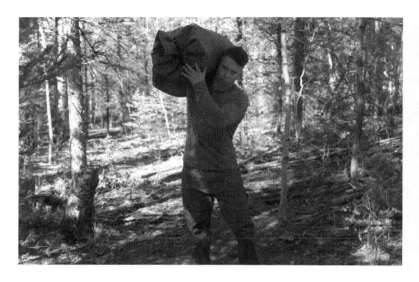

THE SANDBAG SHOULDER CARRY: PROGRAMMING

Finding the correct place in a workout for the shoulder carry can be tricky. The exercise itself is purely strength-based, but getting the sandbag into position requires power. For these reasons, there are two ways to program the movement.

1. Add carries to your last few shoulder attempts of the day. This lets you carry heavier sandbags without taking too much away from your regularly scheduled sandbag-to-shoulder work.
2. Add 1-2 sets of shoulder carries per side near the end of a workout using a lightweight sandbag. Light weight means each set will be longer, so 1-2 sets is all you'll need.

HOLDS, CARRIES, AND PARTIALS

If you're having trouble shouldering a sandbag because of a lack of skill, sometimes the solution is breaking the movement up into smaller parts. For example, if you shoulder sandbags from a vertical starting position on the lap, and you always get stuck three-quarters of the way up the chest, you can bring the sandbag to that spot and hold it there for time.

If you lift from a horizontal position on the lap, and the final bit of rotation from the upper chest to the shoulder is what's holding you back, again bring the sandbag to that spot and keep it there.

You can increase the intensity of these holds by adding movement, turning the exercise into a carry. The idea is to get used to being in those uncomfortable positions.

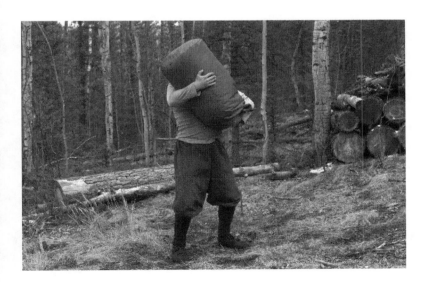

Holds, Carries, and Partials: Programming

If you want to get anything meaningful out of these partial movements they need to be done at a high level of intensity, with complete focus. It will take considerable effort to make those uncomfortable points in the movement less so, therefore these holds or carries should be placed relatively early in the workout, at the beginning of the strength phase.

For best results, perform 3-5 sets of as long as you can manage.

A WEAK PRESS

Unlike the sandbag-to-shoulder, there are no specific sandbag exercises recommended for improving pressing strength. The best way to improve your press is to press more often, both with a sandbag and in your calisthenics workouts.

If you've hit a plateau, you may wish to bias your calisthenics circuit workouts towards vertical pressing movements.

For example, if your workout usually has two pressing movements, a vertical press, and a horizontal press, you might do two vertical presses instead, or change your horizontal pressing movement to a more triceps-focused variation.

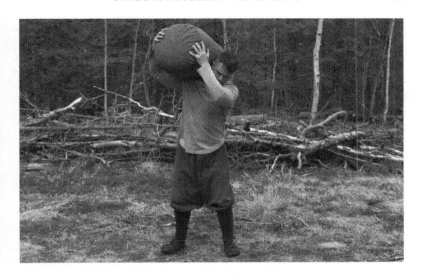

8
CALISTHENICS

YOU COULD BUILD an entire workout program using sandbags and nothing else and come out the other side yoked, strong, and ready.

You could do this and find yourself feeling as powerful as you look, but some things are just too good to pass on. Why settle for exceptional when you can have so much more than that.

There's another training style that blends together so well with heavy sandbag lifting it just has to be here.

It must.

As great as sandbags are alone they pale in comparison to what they become when brought together with their counterpart:

Calisthenics.

Together, sandbags and calisthenics become the perfect form of hybrid training, creating an all-around athlete who's ready for anything and knows it. Strength, power, muscle, endurance, speed, mental fortitude, and a type of total body integrity you don't get any other way will be yours when you combine these training styles.

Every field of exercise has some things it does well, and others it does less well. Every training style leaves gaps somewhere. The primary goal when searching for a complimentary form of exercise to go along with your main focus is to locate those gaps and fill them in. Usually this takes a lot of work, requiring the combining of many different things. Sometimes though, a pairing comes along that fits together so well it creates something truly complete all on its own.

Sandbags and calisthenics are one such pairing.

Sandbags make you a master of moving heavy objects.

Calisthenics makes you a master of moving yourself.

On the surface these two things seem to contradict each other, like they might cancel each other out, but what actually happens is they come together to form the perfect best of both worlds middle place.

In the context of a sandbag-focused program, one form of calisthenics training stands tall above the rest, filling in every possible gap left behind and giving you everything heavy sandbag lifting can't,

The calisthenics circuit.

CALISTHENICS CIRCUITS

Calisthenics circuit training is designed to wear you down quickly and hold you there.

Imagine the final mile of a five-mile run.

You're exhausted, winded, and the only thing driving you forward is sheer power of will.

Now imagine the final mile is full of obstacles.

With four miles already behind you, rather than a simple run to the finish line, you have to make your way up and over things, under things and around them, jumping, crawling, climbing, pushing, bending, calling on strength you didn't know you have from somewhere deep inside yourself, all while fighting the constant reminder playing on repeat in your head, "You still have a long way left to go."

This is what a calisthenics circuit is like, brutal and unrelenting, but well worth the struggle.

While basic on the surface, this training style allows for endless variation and contains within it a great deal of complexity for those who go looking. At its base level, a calisthenics circuit is nothing more than a collection of exercises done back to back for a set number of reps.

Sounds easy enough, right?

That's hardly the half of it.

To make these circuits truly worth your time, you'll be racing the clock. Rather than improving in the normal way by increasing the number of reps you can do in a set, you'll improve by doing the same number of reps in less time.

Your first couple of attempts with a new circuit won't be too bad. More likely than not you'll make significant progress, cutting minutes off your time multiple workouts in a row. Eventually, though, that clock will catch up with you, and you'll need to fight with everything you have for even the smallest improvement.

The well-crafted calisthenics circuit walks a fine line between muscle fatigue and cardio, with the intention of maintaining a perfect balance between the two. In doing so it builds a lot of muscle, keeps you mobile and strong on your feet, builds elite strength endurance, conditioning, and work capacity, and teaches you to push beyond your own perceived limits, giving you a mental toughness far beyond what you could hope to build in any other way, it keeps you lean, and most importantly it does all of these things quickly, without adding excessive fatigue and wearing you down for your heavy sandbag training sessions.

No one circuit will get this balance exactly right for all people, but there are some guidelines you can follow that will help with setting one up.

CREATING A CIRCUIT

Creating something that is equal parts cardio and muscle fatigue is the gold standard of calisthenics circuits. When done right, a balanced circuit will push you all the way to the very edge of both. You'll have just enough strength to complete your reps, and just enough breath left in your lungs to keep pushing towards the end, but not an ounce more than that.

Creating something like this requires careful planning, trial and error, and a great deal of willpower, but once you have it, it's yours to keep, and yours to improve.

The problem with recommending one exact circuit for everyone is that no two people have the exact same strengths and weaknesses, or levels of conditioning. The only way to truly create a circuit that suits you as an individual is to shape it over time. Here are a few guidelines to help you out:

- Use upper body exercises only
- Use 4-5 exercises each focused on a different movement pattern
- Maintain a balance between push and pull
- Circuits should be roughly 20-40 minutes long
- Rotate between 2-3 different circuits

1. USE UPPER BODY EXERCISES ONLY

As tempting as it may be to try doing everything at once, if your goal is building a circuit that balances muscle fatigue and cardio equally, you'll want to leave the lower body out of it.

Pairing upper-body exercises with lower-body exercises will push things way too far in the direction of cardio, and the muscles themselves won't be worked nearly as well. The legs will get all the work they need from lifting heavy sandbags.

2. USE 4-5 EXERCISES EACH FOCUSED ON A DIFFERENT MOVEMENT PATTERN

Upper body movement can be separated into five distinct patterns:

1. Horizontal Push (Push-up variations, dips)
2. Horizontal Pull (Rowing variations)
3. Vertical Push (Pike and handstand push-up variations)
4. Vertical Pull (Pull-up variations)
5. Abdominal Exercises (Technically 'abdominal exercises' is a broad term used to describe many different movement patterns, but grouping them all together here simplifies things.)

If we look at the basic movement patterns of the upper body, each one is focused on a different muscle group (vertical pulling movements primarily work the lats, horizontal pushing movements primarily work the chest, and so on). The trick to crafting a circuit that balances muscle fatigue and cardio equally is allowing for just the right amount of intra-set rest for each muscle group.

Creating a circuit that's made up of one exercise for each pattern does just that.

This setup allows for just enough time between when you do an exercise and when you return to it for some muscle recovery to take place, but not so much recovery that you lose the muscle-building effects that come from staying close to failure.

3. MAINTAIN A BALANCE BETWEEN PUSH AND PULL

A perfect circuit flows seamlessly from one exercise to the next, and back again. You never want to be slowed down because one exercise, or one movement pattern is too difficult compared to the rest.

Individual strengths will play a big part in this, which is why the best circuit for you is one you create yourself, but here's a basic example to get you started:

An Unbalanced Circuit

1. Chin-ups
2. Handstand push-ups
3. Hanging leg raises
4. Inverted rows
5. Dips

In this example, the handstand push-ups are at a much higher difficulty level than the other exercises, and will slow you down. Push and pull are unbalanced. Here are two possible solutions to fix the circuit:

Balanced Circuit One

1. Chin-ups
2. Pike push-ups
3. Hanging leg raises
4. Inverted rows
5. Dips

By replacing the handstand push-ups with pike push-ups, all exercises end up at the same relative difficulty level, and we achieve balance between push and pull.

Balanced Circuit Two

1. Chin-ups
2. Handstand push-ups
3. Hanging leg raises
4. Tuck front lever rows
5. Dips

Rather than making the handstand pushups easier, in this example we make the inverted rows more difficult by replacing them with tuck front lever rows. This also leads to a balance between push and pull, as each side has both a relatively easy exercise and a difficult exercise.

4. CIRCUITS SHOULD BE ROUGHLY 20-40 MINUTES LONG

The goal with these circuits is to increase workout density, to do more work in less time. If a circuit is made up of 200 total reps and takes you 40 minutes to complete, continue working with it until you can finish it in under 20 minutes. Once you reach that 20 minute mark, add more reps to the circuit and start again.

5. ROTATE BETWEEN 2-3 DIFFERENT CIRCUITS

Having a few different circuits you rotate between prevents overuse issues, and allows adaptation to take place at a reasonable pace. Doing the exact same circuit multiple times a week is overkill, and progress will be slow. Too many circuits also means slow progress. Rotating between 2-3 different circuits on a weekly basis will yield the best results.

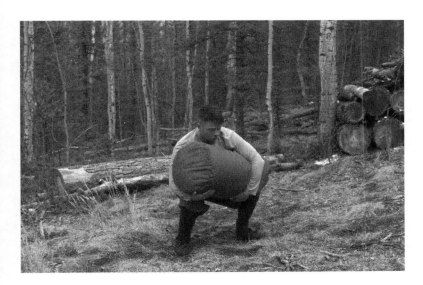

9

PROGRAMS

SANDBAGS & CALISTHENICS BASE PROGRAM

MONDAY

1. Sandbag-to-Shoulder

- 5-15 attempts per side
- 1-2 minutes rest between reps

2. Sandbag High Pull

- 5-10 sets of 3 reps
- 1-2 minutes rest between sets

3. Sandbag Bear Hug Carry

- 3 sets of max distance
- 3-5 minutes rest between sets

4. Lift From the Lap to Chest Height (Vertical Method 1)

- 1 set of max reps

5. Posterior Chain (Band Good Mornings, Bodyweight Hyperextensions, etc.)

- 100 reps

6. Abs (Standing Band Crunches, Sit-ups, etc.)

- 100 reps

7. Obliques (Oblique Crunches etc.)

- 50 reps per side

NOTES:

1. Sandbag-to-Shoulder: Every attempt should start from the ground and end on the shoulder.

2. Sandbag-to-Shoulder & Sandbag High Pulls: Move on when you begin to slow down noticeably, and/or start missing attempts.

3. Sandbag-to-Shoulder: If you can do more than 15 reps per side without slowing down, use a heavier sandbag. If you can't make it past 5 reps, use a lighter sandbag.

4. Posterior Chain, Abs, & Obliques: These exercises should be relatively easy, and shouldn't take more than 10 minutes combined. Use a light band or bodyweight only, and improve by doing your reps more explosively rather than by adding weight.

5. Abs & Obliques: High rep ab exercise is often discredited as unnecessary and ineffective, I disagree. In addition to offering some muscle-building effects, the high rep exercise increases your mind's connection to the muscles in your core, which means a stronger brace. Proper breathing and bracing is essential when lifting heavy sandbags, and anything you can do to improve it is well worth the time investment.

TUESDAY

1. Calisthenics Circuit

- Chin-ups, Dips, Inverted Rows, Pike Push-ups, Ab Wheel Rollouts
- '10 Down' rep scheme

2. Neck Curls & Extensions

- 4 sets of 25 reps each

3. Optional Isolation Work

- 10 minutes maximum

NOTES:

1. 10 Down: A '10 Down' rep scheme is 10 reps of each exercise, then 9 of each, 8 of each, all the way down to 1 rep of each exercise.

(10, 9, 8, 7, 6, 5, 4, 3, 2, 1)

2. Calisthenics Circuit: Set a timer at the start of the workout and complete the circuit as fast as you're able while maintaining proper exercise technique. When you're able to complete the circuit in under 20 minutes, switch to a '10 Down and Up' rep scheme.

(10, 9, 8, 7, 6, 5, 4, 3, 2, 1, 1, 2, 3, 4, 5, 6, 7, 8, 9, 10)

3. Neck Training: The 4 sets of 25 includes warm up sets. Each set should be progressively heavier until the final all-out set of 25.

4. Optional Isolation Work: Every muscle will grow from this program as is. You don't need any additional isolation work. That said, if you have any specific muscle groups you want to isolate (arms, shoulders, calves etc.), here's where you'll do it. Make sure to follow these rules:

1. Nothing Heavy. The last thing you want to do during this time is heavy deadlifts. Stick to lightweight isolation movements for small muscle groups.

2. Cap this part of the workout at 10 minutes. Any more and recovery will be compromised.

WEDNESDAY

Off

THURSDAY

1. Sandbag-to-Shoulder

- 5-15 attempts per side
- 1-2 minutes rest between reps

2. Sandbag Row

- 5-10 sets of 3 reps
- 1-2 minutes rest between sets

3. Sandbag Squat

- 3 sets of 5-20 reps
- 3-5 minutes rest between sets

4. Lift From the Lap to Chest Height (Horizontal High Lift)

- 1 set of max reps

5. Posterior Chain (Band Good Mornings, Body-weight Hyperextensions etc.)

* 100 reps

6. Abs (Standing Band Crunches, Sit-ups etc.)

* 100 reps

7. Obliques (Oblique Crunches etc.)

* 50 reps per side

NOTES:

Sandbag Row: Move on if your form begins to break down.

FRIDAY

1. Calisthenics Circuit

* Wide Grip Pull-ups, Decline Deficit Pike Push-ups, Hanging Leg Raises, Ring Rows, Dive-bomber Push-ups
* '5-3-2' rep scheme (5 rounds)

2. Neck Curls & Extensions

- 4 sets of 25 reps each

3. Optional Isolation Work

- 10 minutes maximum

NOTES:

5-3-2 Rep Scheme: Complete 5 reps of each exercise, followed by 3 reps of each, and finally 2 reps of each. This is one round. When you manage to complete all rounds in under 20 minutes, add more.

SATURDAY/SUNDAY

Off

SANDBAGS & CALISTHENICS BASE PROGRAM NOTES

1. Five-Week Cycle: This program is meant to be run in 5-week cycles. Complete the entire week-long program 4 weeks in a row, and take the 5th week off to deload.

2. Deload Week: Either take the entire week off completely or give yourself three, 30-minute sessions during the week to work on something unrelated to sandbags and calisthenics, just nothing too overly taxing. Hiking, swimming, riding a bike, or working on your mobility are good examples, lifting a heavy barbell is not.

3. Heavy Sandbag Lifting: Heavy sandbag lifting forces you to tap into a state of mind you don't normally use in daily life, a state of raw, life-or-death-like aggression. For some individuals the ability to reach this state becomes more difficult without frequent use. For this reason your first workout back after the week-long deload might not be your best. Weights will feel heavier, and the power you spent so long building might seem out of reach. This is normal. Push through that first workout, and you'll come back next time stronger than ever.

4. Moving Forward: Over the course of the 5-week cycle, use the sandbag-to-shoulder as a guide to determine your weak point. There are three main weak points when trying to shoulder a sandbag: from the ground, from the lap to chest height, and from chest height to the shoulder. For each of these weak points, I've created a unique, 5-week training program for you to follow. In this way, you can link together 5-week training cycles indefinitely, strengthening any weak points as they turn up.

For example, if the most difficult part of shouldering a sandbag during the first 5-week base program is moving the sandbag from your upper chest to your shoulder, you'll move on to the 'Sandbags & Calisthenics Base Program Variation Three: Weak From Chest to Shoulder' program. After that 5-week cycle you may wish to repeat it, or move on to a different 5-week cycle focused on something else. It's not uncommon to run the same program multiple times in a row. If you're not sure which program to run next, return to the base program until a new weak point makes itself known.

5. Calisthenics Circuits: The calisthenics circuits outlined in the program are there as examples, and you may need to change them based on your own abilities. If chin-ups are too difficult, replace them with something else. If basic pike push-ups are too easy, elevate your feet. The exact exercises aren't important. Follow the guidelines from the chapter on creating a calisthenics circuit, train hard, and you will see results.

SANDBAGS & CALISTHENICS BASE PROGRAM VARIATION ONE: WEAK OFF THE GROUND

MONDAY

1. One-Motion Ground to Chest (Horizontal or Standing Upright)

- 5 single reps
- 1-2 minutes rest between reps

2. Sandbag-to-Shoulder

- 5-15 attempts per side
- 1-2 minutes rest between reps

3. Sandbag High Pull

- 5 sets of 3 reps
- 1-2 minutes rest between sets

4. Sandbag Bear Hug Carry

- 3 sets of max distance
- 3-5 minutes rest between sets

5. Lift From the Lap to Chest Height (Vertical Method 1)

- 1 set of max reps

6. Posterior Chain (Band Good Mornings, Body-weight Hyperextensions etc.)

- 100 reps

7. Abs (Standing Band Crunches, Sit-ups etc.)

- 100 reps

8. Obliques (Oblique Crunches etc.)

- 50 reps per side

TUESDAY

1. Calisthenics Circuit

- Neutral Pull-ups, Plyometric Push-ups, Inverted Rows, Decline Pike Push-ups, Ab Wheel Rollouts

- 'I o Down' rep scheme

2. Neck Curls & Extensions

- 4 sets of 25 reps each

3. Optional Isolation Work

- I o minutes maximum

WEDNESDAY

Off

THURSDAY

1. One-Motion Ground to Chest (Horizontal or Standing Upright)

- 5 single reps
- I-2 minutes rest between reps

2. Sandbag-to-Shoulder

- 5-I 5 attempts per side
- I-2 minutes rest between reps

3. Sandbag Row

- 5 sets of 3 reps
- 1-2 minutes rest between sets

4. Sandbag Box Squat (Sandbag in Horizontal Position)

- 3 sets of 5-20 reps
- 3-5 minutes rest between sets

5. Posterior Chain (Band Good Mornings, Bodyweight Hyperextensions etc.)

- 100 reps

6. Abs (Standing Band Crunches, Sit-ups etc.)

- 100 reps

7. Obliques (Oblique Crunches etc.)

- 50 reps per side

FRIDAY

1. Calisthenics Circuit

- Pull-ups, Decline Diamond Push-ups, Ab Wheel Rollouts, Deficit Push-ups
- '10 Down and Up' rep scheme

2. Neck Curls & Extensions

- 4 sets of 25 reps each

3. Optional Isolation Work

- 10 minutes maximum

NOTES:

10 Down and Up: If you're able to complete the full '10 down and up' circuit in under 20 minutes, switch to a '10 down and up and down' and so on.

SATURDAY/SUNDAY

Off

SANDBAGS & CALISTHENICS BASE PROGRAM VARIATION TWO: WEAK OFF THE LAP

MONDAY

1. Sandbag-to-Shoulder

- 5-15 attempts per side
- 1-2 minutes rest between reps

2. Sandbag High Pull

- 5-10 sets of 3 reps
- 1-2 minutes rest between sets

3. Sandbag Bear Hug Carry

- 3 sets of max distance
- 3-5 minutes rest between sets

4. Lift From the Lap to Chest Height (Vertical Method 1)

- 1 set of max reps

5. Posterior Chain (Band Good Mornings, Body-weight Hyperextensions etc.)

- 100 reps

6. Abs (Standing Band Crunches, Sit-ups etc.)

- 100 reps

7. Obliques (Oblique Crunches etc.)

- 50 reps per side

TUESDAY

1. Calisthenics Circuit

- L-Sit Chin-ups, Dips, Ring Rows, Divebomber Push-ups, Ab Wheel Rollouts
- '10 Down' rep scheme

2. Neck Curls & Extensions

- 4 sets of 25 reps each

3. Optional Isolation Work

- 10 minutes maximum

WEDNESDAY

Off

THURSDAY

1. Sandbag-to-Shoulder

- 5-15 attempts per side
- 1-2 minutes rest between reps

2. Lift From The Lap to Chest Height (Vertical Method 2)

- 5 sets of 3 reps
- 1-2 minutes rest between sets

3. Sandbag Box Squat (Sandbag in Vertical Position)

- 5 sets of 3 reps
- 1-2 minutes rest between sets

4. Lift From The Lap to Chest Height (Horizontal High Lift)

- 1 set max reps

5. Posterior Chain (Band Good Mornings, Bodyweight Hyperextensions etc.)

- 100 reps

6. Abs (Standing Band Crunches, Sit-ups etc.)

- 100 reps

7. Obliques (Oblique Crunches etc.)

- 50 reps per side

FRIDAY

1. Calisthenics Circuit

- Pull-ups, Decline Pike Push-ups, Hanging Leg Raises, Inverted Rows, Decline Diamond Push-ups
- '10 Down and Up' rep scheme

2. Neck Curls & Extensions

- 4 sets of 25 reps each

3. Optional Isolation Work

- 10 minutes maximum

SATURDAY/SUNDAY

Off

SANDBAGS & CALISTHENICS BASE PROGRAM VARIATION THREE: WEAK FROM CHEST TO SHOULDER

MONDAY

1. Sandbag-to-Shoulder

- 5-15 attempts per side
- 1-2 minutes rest between reps

2. Sandbag High Pull

- 5-10 sets of 3 reps
- 1-2 minutes rest between sets

3. Carry With Sandbag Held at Weak Point

- 3 sets of max distance
- 3-5 minutes rest between sets

4. Lift From the Lap to Chest Height (Vertical Method 1)

- 1 set of max reps

5. Posterior Chain (Band Good Mornings, Bodyweight Hyperextensions etc.)

- 100 reps

6. Abs (Standing Band Crunches, Sit-ups etc.)

- 100 reps

7. Obliques (Oblique Crunches etc.)

- 50 reps per side

TUESDAY

1. Calisthenics Circuit

- Wide Grip Pull-ups, Dips, Ring Rows, Plyometric Push-ups, Ab Wheel Rollouts
- '6-5-4' rep scheme (4 rounds)

2. Neck Curls & Extensions

- 4 sets of 25 reps each

3. Optional Isolation Work

- 10 minutes maximum

WEDNESDAY

Off

THURSDAY

1. Sandbag-to-Shoulder

- 5-15 attempts per side
- 1-2 minutes rest between reps

2. Sandbag Shoulder Carry

- Done as part of the last two sandbag-to-shoulder attempts per side for the day (4 total carries)
- 4 sets of max distance

3. Carry With Sandbag Held at Weak Point

- 3 sets of max distance
- 3-5 minutes rest between sets

4. Sandbag Box Squat (Sandbag Held in Horizontal Position)

- 1 set max reps

5. Posterior Chain (Band Good Mornings, Bodyweight Hyperextensions etc.)

- 100 reps

6. Abs (Standing Band Crunches, Sit-ups etc.)

- 100 reps

7. Obliques (Oblique Crunches etc.)

- 50 reps per side

FRIDAY

1. Calisthenics Circuit

- Chin-ups, Pike Push-ups, Hanging Leg Raises, Inverted Rows, Diamond Push-ups
- '15 down' rep scheme

2. Neck Curls & Extensions

- 4 sets of 25 reps each

3. Optional Isolation Work

- 10 minutes maximum

SATURDAY/SUNDAY

Off

SANDBAGS & CALISTHENICS ALTERNATE PROGRAM

MONDAY (A)

1. Sandbag Push Press

- 5-15 attempts
- 1-2 minutes rest between reps

2. Sandbag-to-Shoulder

- 5-10 attempts per side
- 1-2 minutes rest between reps

3. Sandbag Press

- 3 sets of 5-20 reps
- 3-5 minutes rest between sets

4. Sandbag Box Squat (Sandbag Held in Vertical Position)

- 1 set of max reps

5. Posterior Chain (Band Good Mornings, Bodyweight Hyperextensions etc.)

- 100 reps

6. Abs (Standing Band Crunches, Sit-ups etc.)

- 100 reps

7. Obliques (Oblique Crunches etc.)

- 50 reps per side

NOTES:

1. Sandbag Push Press: Move on when form breaks down, and/or when you start missing attempts.

TUESDAY

1. Calisthenics Circuit

- Chin-ups, Dips, Inverted Rows, Pike Push-ups, Ab Wheel Rollouts
- '10 Down' rep scheme

2. Neck Curls & Extensions

- 4 sets of 25 reps each

3. Optional Isolation Work

- 10 minutes maximum

WEDNESDAY (B)

1. Sandbag-to-Shoulder

- 5-15 attempts per side
- 1-2 minutes rest between reps

2. Sandbag High Pull

- 5-10 sets of 3 reps
- 1-2 minutes rest between sets

3. Sandbag Bear Hug Carry

- 3 sets of max distance
- 3-5 minutes rest between sets

4. Sandbag Press

- 3 sets of 5-20 reps
- 3-5 minutes rest between sets

5. Posterior Chain (Band Good Mornings, Body-weight Hyperextensions etc.)

- 100 reps

6. Abs (Standing Band Crunches, Sit-ups etc.)

- 100 reps

7. Obliques (Oblique Crunches etc.)

- 50 reps per side

THURSDAY

Off

FRIDAY (A)

1. Sandbag Push Press

- 5-15 attempts
- 1-2 minutes rest between reps

2. Sandbag-to-Shoulder

- 5-10 attempts per side
- 1-2 minutes rest between reps

3. Sandbag Press

- 3 sets of 5-20 reps
- 3-5 minutes rest between sets

4. Sandbag Box Squat (Sandbag Held in Vertical Position)

- 1 set of max reps

5. Posterior Chain (Band Good Mornings, Bodyweight Hyperextensions etc.)

- 100 reps

6. Abs (Standing Band Crunches, Sit-ups etc.)

- 100 reps

7. Obliques (Oblique Crunches etc.)

- 50 reps per side

SATURDAY

1. Calisthenics Circuit

- Wide Grip Pull-ups, Decline Deficit Pike Push-ups, Hanging Leg Raises, Ring Rows, Divebomber Push-ups
- '5-3-2' rep scheme (5 rounds)

2. Neck Curls & Extensions

- 4 sets of 25 reps each

3. Optional Isolation Work

- 10 minutes maximum

SUNDAY

Off

SANDBAGS & CALISTHENICS ALTERNATE PROGRAM NOTES

1. A, B, A: In this program, you will rotate between two different sandbag training days. In week one, Monday is workout A, Wednesday is workout B, and Friday is workout A again. In Week two, Monday is workout B, Wednesday is workout A, and Friday is workout B again, and so on.

2. Five-Week Cycle: This program follows the same 5 week cycle and progression model outlined in the 'Sandbags & Calisthenics Base Program'.

3. Weak Off The Lap: This base version of the 'Sandbags & Calisthenics Alternate Program' is already focused on building strength off the lap. If lifting a sandbag from the lap is your weak point, repeat this 5-week cycle again.

SANDBAGS & CALISTHENICS ALTERNATE PROGRAM VARIATION ONE: WEAK OFF THE GROUND

MONDAY (A)

1. Sandbag Push Press

- 5-15 attempts

- 1-2 minutes rest between reps

2. One-Motion Ground to Chest (Horizontal or Standing Upright)

- 5 single reps
- 1-2 minutes rest between reps

3. Sandbag-to-Shoulder

- 5-10 attempts per side
- 1-2 minutes rest between reps

4. Sandbag Row

- 5-10 sets of 3 reps
- 1-2 minutes rest between sets

5. Sandbag Press

- 3 sets of 5-20 reps
- 3-5 minutes rest between sets

6. Posterior Chain (Band Good Mornings, Body-weight Hyperextensions etc.)

- 100 reps

7. Abs (Standing Band Crunches, Sit-ups etc.)

- 100 reps

8. Obliques (Oblique Crunches etc.)

- 50 reps per side

TUESDAY

1. Calisthenics Circuit

- Neutral Pull-ups, Plyometric Push-ups, Inverted
  Rows, Decline Pike Push-ups, Ab Wheel Rollouts
- '10 Down' rep scheme

2. Neck Curls & Extensions

- 4 sets of 25 reps each

3. Optional Isolation Work

- 10 minutes maximum

WEDNESDAY (B)

1. One-Motion Ground to Chest (Horizontal or Standing Upright)

- 5 single reps
- 1-2 minutes rest between reps

2. Sandbag-to-Shoulder

- 5-15 attempts per side
- 1-2 minutes rest between reps

3. Sandbag High Pull

- 5-10 sets of 3 reps
- 1-2 minutes rest between sets

4. Sandbag Bear Hug Carry

- 3 sets of max distance
- 3-5 minutes rest between sets

5. Sandbag Press

- 3 sets of 5-20 reps
- 3-5 minutes rest between sets

6. Posterior Chain (Band Good Mornings, Body-weight Hyperextensions etc.)

- 100 reps

7. Abs (Standing Band Crunches, Sit-ups etc.)

- 100 reps

8. Obliques (Oblique Crunches etc.)

- 50 reps per side

THURSDAY

Off

FRIDAY (A)

1. Sandbag Push Press

- 5-15 attempts
- 1-2 minutes rest between reps

2. One-Motion Ground to Chest (Horizontal or Standing Upright)

- 5 single reps
- 1-2 minutes rest between reps

3. Sandbag-to-Shoulder

- 5-10 attempts per side
- 1-2 minutes rest between reps

4. Sandbag Row

- 5-10 sets of 3 reps

- 1-2 minutes rest between sets

5. Sandbag Press

- 3 sets of 5-20 reps
- 3-5 minutes rest between sets

6. Posterior Chain (Band Good Mornings, Body-weight Hyperextensions etc.)

- 100 reps

7. Abs (Standing Band Crunches, Sit-ups etc.)

- 100 reps

8. Obliques (Oblique Crunches etc.)

- 50 reps per side

SATURDAY

1. Calisthenics Circuit

- Pull-ups, Decline Diamond Push-ups, Ab Wheel Rollouts, Deficit Push-ups
- '10 Down and Up' rep scheme

2. Neck Curls & Extensions

- 4 sets of 25 reps each

3. Optional Isolation Work

- 10 minutes maximum

SUNDAY

Off

SANDBAGS & CALISTHENICS ALTERNATE PROGRAM VARIATION TWO: WEAK FROM CHEST TO SHOULDER

MONDAY (A)

1. Sandbag Push Press

- 5-15 attempts
- 1-2 minutes rest between reps

2. Sandbag-to-Shoulder

- 5-10 attempts per side
- 1-2 minutes rest between reps

3. Carry With Sandbag Held at Weak Point

- 3 sets of max distance
- 3-5 minutes rest between sets

4. Sandbag Press

- 3 sets of 5-20 reps
- 3-5 minutes rest between sets

5. Posterior Chain (Band Good Mornings, Bodyweight Hyperextensions etc.)

- 100 reps

6. Abs (Standing Band Crunches, Sit-ups etc.)

- 100 reps

7. Obliques (Oblique Crunches etc.)

- 50 reps per side

TUESDAY

1. Calisthenics Circuit

- Wide Grip Pull-ups, Dips, Ring Rows, Plyometric Push-ups, Ab Wheel Rollouts
- '6-5-4' rep scheme (4 rounds)

2. Neck Curls & Extensions

- 4 sets of 25 reps each

3. Optional Isolation Work

- 10 minutes maximum

WEDNESDAY (B)

1. Sandbag-to-Shoulder

- 5-15 attempts per side
- 1-2 minutes rest between reps

2. Shoulder Carry

- Done as part of the last two sandbag-to-shoulder attempts per side for the day (4 total carries)
- 4 sets of max distance

3. Sandbag High Pull

- 5-10 sets of 3 reps
- 1-2 minutes rest between sets

4. Sandbag Press

- 3 sets of 5-20 reps
- 3-5 minutes rest between sets

5. Posterior Chain (Band Good Mornings, Bodyweight Hyperextensions etc.)

- 100 reps

6. Abs (Standing Band Crunches, Sit-ups etc.)

- 100 reps

7. Obliques (Oblique Crunches etc.)

- 50 reps per side

THURSDAY

Off

FRIDAY (A)

1. Sandbag Push Press

- 5-15 attempts
- 1-2 minutes rest between reps

2. Sandbag-to-Shoulder

- 5-10 attempts per side
- 1-2 minutes rest between reps

3. Carry With Sandbag Held at Weak Point

- 3 sets of max distance

- 3-5 minutes rest between sets

4. Sandbag Press

- 3 sets of 5-20 reps
- 3-5 minutes rest between sets

5. Posterior Chain (Band Good Mornings, Body-weight Hyperextensions etc.)

- 100 reps

6. Abs (Standing Band Crunches, Sit-ups etc.)

- 100 reps

7. Obliques (Oblique Crunches etc.)

- 50 reps per side

SATURDAY

1. Calisthenics Circuit

- Chin-ups, Pike Push-ups, Hanging Leg Raises, Inverted Rows, Diamond Push-ups
- '15 down' rep scheme

2. Neck Curls & Extensions

- 4 sets of 25 reps each

3. Optional Isolation Work

- 10 minutes maximum

SUNDAY

Off

ABOUT THE AUTHOR

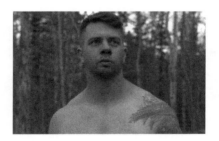

Cody Janko, also known as 'The Stone Circle' on YouTube is a certified personal trainer, the owner of a rescue dog focused animal care business, and fan of all things fitness. When he's not wandering the mountain forests in his medieval garb searching for rocks to lift, you're likely to find him sitting at home with his two dogs Clover and Cash, reading fantasy books or working on his next video. Follow Cody here:

Made in the USA
Middletown, DE
10 September 2024

60671708R00091